THE *NEW*
ATKINS
FOR A NEW YOU
WORKBOOK

A WEEKLY FOOD JOURNAL to HELP YOU
SHED WEIGHT and FEEL GREAT

Colette Heimowitz

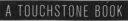
A TOUCHSTONE BOOK
Published by Simon & Schuster
New York   London   Toronto   Sydney   New Delhi

D0047887

Touchstone
A Division of Simon & Schuster, Inc.
1230 Avenue of the Americas
New York, NY 10020

Copyright © 2012 by Atkins Nutritionals, Inc.

First Touchstone trade paperback edition December 2012

TOUCHSTONE and colophon are registered trademarks of
Simon & Schuster, Inc.

For information about special discounts for bulk purchases,
please contact Simon & Schuster Special Sales at 1-866-506-1949
or business@simonandschuster.com.

The Simon & Schuster Speakers Bureau can bring authors
to your live event. For more information or to book an event,
contact the Simon & Schuster Speakers Bureau at 866-248-3049
or visit our website at www.simonspeakers.com.

Designed by Ruth Lee-Mui

Manufactured in the United States of America

10 9 8 7 6 5 4 3 2 1

ISBN 978-1-4767-1557-5
ISBN 978-1-4767-1558-2 (ebook)

ALSO FROM ATKINS

The New Atkins for a New You

The New Atkins for a New You Cookbook

CONTENTS

GETTING STARTED

Welcome to *The New Atkins for a New You Workbook*. Like most people, you probably have a lot on your plate and only so many hours each day to accomplish that daunting to-do list. Keeping track of your diet may seem like the last thing you have time for. Not to worry; this 16-week journal, a companion to the bestselling books *The New Atkins for a New You* and *The New Atkins for a New You Cookbook*, will make it easy to do. Which in turn will make it easier to reach your weight goals—even as you stay on top of your work and family responsibilities, too. Soon you'll be one of the millions of people who have lost weight on the Atkins Diet.

WHY A WORKBOOK?

The evidence is pretty conclusive that keeping a food journal detailing one's progress increases the likelihood of weight-loss success. For example, in a 2008 study at Kaiser Permanente's Center for Health Research involving almost 1,700 people, those who kept a food diary lost twice as much weight as participants who didn't record their meals.

So why sixteen weeks? The research on habit formation is less clear cut. A person's personality and level of commitment play a huge role in her ability to change her behavior, as does the type of habit. Developing a simple habit, such as eating a piece of fruit every day or having a glass of water every two hours, is obviously easier to achieve than one that requires greater commitment, such as walking four miles a day or changing the long-standing eating habits necessary to slim down. As a nutritionist, I've found that it takes most people at least twelve weeks, and often closer to sixteen weeks, to establish new eating habits. Four months should also allow most people with a moderate amount of weight to lose, say 30 pounds, enough time to achieve or get close to their goal. Even if you reach your desired weight before 16 weeks, it's important to continue to record your meals and other behavior. Why? Because Atkins is not just a weight-loss diet but also a permanent way of eating; you'll want to establish the level of carb intake that will let you maintain your new weight.

This workbook combines the Atkins track record of safe and reliable weight loss without feeling hungry and deprived with the power of journaling to boost your motivation and therefore the likelihood that you'll be able to take off those unwanted pounds and inches—fast—and keep them off.

ATKINS 101

Atkins is a low-carbohydrate diet, which means you don't have to count calories. Instead, you track grams of carbs, specifically Net Carbs (see "What Are Net Carbs?" on page 3). The low-quality, high-sugar carbs that dominate the standard American diet are more quickly converted to glucose than fiber-rich carbs. As long as you eat lots of carb foods, particularly those that are quickly metabolized, there's never any need to resort to your fat stores for energy. Fat remains on your abdomen, hips, buttocks, and thighs. That's why it's so hard to lose weight on a conventional low-fat diet, unless your calorie intake is superlow, leaving you constantly hungry. Not surprisingly, most people find this weight-loss approach unsustainable and quickly revert to their old way of eating.

Atkins is different. It enables you to simply use your backup energy supply, fat, as your primary energy source instead of glucose from carbs, much as a hybrid car runs on either gasoline or electricity. This is hardly a new concept: This dual system allowed our forebears to survive when food was scarce by burning their body fat. Your body will always burn glucose and glycogen first, but once they're used up, it turns naturally to fat, including on your hips and abdomen, as an energy source.

WHAT ARE NET CARBS?

Net Carbs are digestible carbs or nonimpact carbs, meaning they exclude the grams of fiber found in many carbohydrate foods. Although fiber is technically a carbohydrate, it doesn't metabolize the way other carbs do and therefore has no impact on your blood sugar level. Most carb counters, including the abridged version in this workbook (see pages 298–324, or for a more complete version, download www.atkins.com/Program/Carb-Counter.aspx), provide Net Carbs for most common foods. To calculate the Net Carbs in packaged foods, simply subtract the number of grams of dietary fiber (and, in the case of low-carb foods, sugar alcohols—a type of low-calorie sweetener) from the total number of carbohydrate grams in a serving. (This information is found on the package's Nutritional Facts panel).

That's why natural fats such as olive oil, butter, sour cream, and avocado, along with eggs, chicken, fish, lamb, beef, pork, and nuts (after the first two weeks), all of which contain fats, are on the Atkins menu. As long as you're burning these healthy natural fats for energy (along with excess body fat) by keeping your carb intake low, they're not depositing fat on your tummy or thighs or clogging your arteries. I call this process flipping the metabolic switch. For more on how Atkins works, read *The New Atkins for a New You* or visit www.atkins.com.

A FOUR-PHASE PROGRAM

The sequential phases of the Atkins Diet are designed to allow you to gradually reintroduce more carbohydrates into your diet, as you also broaden your carb food choices. This way you'll come to understand your overall tolerance for carbs and whether certain foods trigger undue hunger and cravings that could sabotage your forward momentum. You'll achieve your initial objective, jump-starting weight loss in Phase 1, Induction, by eating carbs primarily in the form of vegetables, along with moderate amounts of protein and healthy, natural fats. (With the exception of oils and sugars, most foods contain two or more of the macronutrients fat, protein, and carbohydrates. For simplicity's sake, we'll refer to carbohydrate, protein, or fat foods when that macronutrient predominates.) As you move forward you'll incorporate more nutrient-rich carbohydrate foods such as berries and whole grains, while continuing to steadily shed pounds.

Most people spend at least two weeks in Phase 1, Induction, before moving on to Phase 2, Ongoing Weight Loss (OWL). There you'll begin to discover your personal daily tolerance for carbs, meaning the number of grams of Net Carbs you can consume each day while continuing to lose weight. We recommend that you lose your final 10 pounds in Phase 3, Pre-Maintenance, where you'll also stabilize your new weight, by finding the number of daily grams of Net Carbs you can consume and *maintain* your weight. That way, by the time you've reached your goal weight, you'll know exactly how many grams of Net Carbs and what foods you can consume each day. Finally, you'll move on to Phase 4, Lifetime Maintenance, which becomes your permanent way of eating. To learn which foods you eat in each phase, see "What You Can Eat When" on page 21.

JUST HOW FAST CAN I LOSE WEIGHT?

People who adhere to the new Atkins Diet can lose up to 15 pounds in the first two weeks. Ladies, that can translate into one or two clothing sizes; guys, you'll likely be able to tighten your belt a few notches as that belly recedes. With these results you'll be super-motivated to stay with the program. Another powerful motivator is that you'll be eating healthful food—that's *real* food with *real* flavor in *real-life* portions. Think veggies sautéed in olive oil; grilled chicken, fish, or beef; a mixed greens or spinach salad tossed with creamy blue cheese dressing; a cheese omelet garnished with avocado and cherry tomatoes; and even cream in your coffee or tea. Once you're in Phase 2, Ongoing Weight Loss, you can also savor blueberries, strawberries, cantaloupe, and other low-glycemic fruits.

Of course, we're all different. You may lose more or less than 15 pounds in the first two weeks, or you may lose fewer pounds but find that your clothes fit better as you lose inches. (That's why your measurements are as important as your weight as a tracking device.) Obviously, the more compliant you are, the more likely you are to see impressive results. Likewise, being physically active works in tandem with controlling your carb intake. And the heavier you are, the faster the initial weight drops.

Then there are a number of factors you can't control, like whether you have a sluggish metabolism or a fast one; or even whether you were born male or female. (Guys do have the advantage here.) Younger people also have an easier time losing excess pounds and inches than do older folks. Health or hormonal issues can slow you down as well. But know this: All things being equal, research shows that when compared to traditional calorie- and fat-restricted diets, Atkins consistently does as well as or even outperforms other weight-loss programs.

BACKED BY SCIENCE

The last few years have seen an explosion in the number of studies on why we gain weight (and regain it after losing it), the health risks associated with excess pounds, and the factors that enable weight loss. More than sixty clinical studies have demonstrated that the low-carb lifestyle is a safe and extremely effective way to lose weight and keep it off. The research also makes it crystal clear that controlling carb intake, avoiding added sugars, and eating plenty of nutrient-rich and fiber-rich vegetables along with healthy natural fats and a moderate amount of protein are the ticket to minimizing the blood sugar imbalances that drive cravings for the very foods that cause them—and that can lead to type 2 diabetes. You'll also likely see improved blood pressure readings, lower triglycerides, and other heart health indicator improvements.

WHY DOES ATKINS WORK?

You shift your metabolism. By eliminating sugary treats, starchy snack foods, beverages full of high-fructose corn syrup, bread made with refined white flour and other such foods, you'll change how your body metabolizes food to create energy. The standard American diet (SAD) is high in carbohydrates (carbs), which quickly convert to blood sugar (glucose), which provides the energy for your body's myriad functions, including chasing after your kids, playing tennis, or just moving from here to there. Most of that glucose is converted to fat. That's right, the carbs create body fat. The only way to get rid of that fat is to burn it for energy, which is what happens when you control your carb intake.

You aren't hungry. In the most basic terms, when you change the balance of fats, protein, and carbs in your diet, your body responds differently. Eliminate empty carbs—think sugar, refined flour and other grains, beverages made with high-fructose corn syrup, and most processed foods—and eat primarily whole-food carbs such as vegetables, and there's no need to be obsessed with dietary fat. In fact, natural fats provide satiety, the comfortable feeling of fullness, which helps you control your appetite. Fat also carries satisfying flavor, another reason why you won't find yourself "grazing" shortly after a meal. On Atkins, you needn't starve yourself to see results; in fact, you can have two snacks a day if you wish. And when you're not consumed with hunger, there's no reason to overeat.

Weight comes off fast. The result is speedy weight loss without cravings. And the first pounds and inches that disappear are around your waist and tummy, the very excess weight that puts you at greater risk for type 2 diabetes and other diseases. Rapid weight loss is tremendously motivating, making it easy to stay with the program.

HOW DO I BEGIN?

Weigh in and measure up. Knowing your starting point will also help you establish realistic goals and a time frame in which to achieve them. Note your current weight and several key measurements—you'll find them in the journal—and jot down the time of day. If possible, it's best to weigh and measure yourself at the same time of day.

See your doctor. You should check in with your physician before beginning any weight-loss program. He or she will also check your blood sugar and blood pressure levels, as well as order some tests, including a lipid panel (total, HDL ["good"], and LDL ["bad"] cholesterol, and triglycerides). Once you slim down—or after three to six months on the program—you'll want to have these tests redone. Almost certainly, you'll see improvements on all fronts, which will motivate you to make Atkins your permanent way of eating. If you have type 2 diabetes, see "Diabetics, Take Note." You may need to discuss other drug dosage adjustments as well.

DIABETICS, TAKE NOTE

If you have diabetes, doing Atkins will naturally reduce your blood sugar level, necessitating a reduction in your blood sugar-lowering medication or insulin dosage. Talk to your physician before you begin, track your blood sugar readings faithfully, and stay in touch with him or her as you see those readings change. You'll likely be told to adjust your dosage, but never do so without your physician's guidance.

Evaluate your body composition. There are two simple gauges of body composition, and therefore fitness, to compute before you begin. These numbers may play a role in helping you decide in which phase of Atkins to begin and you can track them and see tangible improvement as you slim down. Your body mass index (BMI) is the traditional gauge of overweight or obesity, but equally important is your waist-to-hip ratio (WHR). People who are "apple shaped," meaning they carry excess pounds around their middle, tend to have more weight-related health issues than those who are "pear shaped," with excess pounds around the hips.

FIND YOUR BODY MASS INDEX

The BMI roughly determines your body composition by calculating the ratio of your weight to your height. However, the BMI doesn't take into consideration your bone density, build, body shape, gender, and age. As a result, individuals who are extremely muscular could have a BMI that suggests that they're overweight despite having very little body fat. Regardless of its shortcomings, the BMI offers clues about whether your weight is within a healthy range, as follows:

Underweight: BMI of <18.5
Normal: BMI of 18.5–24.9
Overweight: BMI of 25–29.9
Obese: BMI of 30 or greater

To find your BMI, enter your height and weight into the calculator on the Atkins website (www.atkins.com/Free-Tools.aspx). Or multiply your weight in pounds by 703 and then divide by your height in inches squared. For example, if you're five feet, six inches tall, and weigh 155 pounds: 108,965 (155 x 703) ÷ 4356 = 25.

Select the phase in which to begin. Deciding how many pounds you want to shed and determining your BMI and WHR are important tools in determining which phase of the Atkins Diet to begin with. Generally, the larger the amount of weight and the higher your BMI and/or the lower your WHR, the earlier the phase you should choose because the lower carb count will kick-start weight loss and hasten progress. (Go to atkins.com/Free-Tools.aspx for a BMI calculator, which will also suggest which phase would be best to start with.) Most people with 30 or more pounds to lose start in Phase 1, Induction. With less than 15 pounds to lose as your goal, starting in Phase 2 is an option if you're willing to swap slower weight loss for more food options. However, you can start in any phase that feels right to you and change your mind at any time.

FIND YOUR WAIST-TO-HIP RATIO

This indicator is a simple matter of comparing the circumference of your waist to that of your hips. Measure yourself nude or in your underwear. Start with the narrowest part of your waist. If you have no discernible indentation at your waist, measure yourself one inch above your navel. Measure your hips at the widest point of your buttocks, usually about nine inches below your waist. To find your WHR, divide the measurement of your waist by the measurement of your hips. If, for example, a woman's waist is 33 and her hips are 38, her WHR would be 0.87. If a man's waist is 38 and his hips are 40, his WHR would be 0.95.

The World Health Organization (WHO) states that a healthy WHR for a woman is 0.85 or below, although a ratio of 0.70 is generally regarded as ideal. That means our hypothetical woman above is considered to be at a health risk. Men's hips are generally narrower than women's, so a man is not considered overweight unless his ratio is 0.90 or above. The hypothetical man cited above has an optimal ratio. Other health organizations may use slightly different parameters. An epidemiological study, *Interheart*, published in the Lancet, states that there is increased risk of disease with a WHR of more than 0.80 in women and 0.95 in men.

CAN I PERSONALIZE THE PROGRAM?

Of course you can. "The Phases Decoded" in page 19 describes the way most people do Atkins, but you can make numerous modifications depending upon your metabolism, lifestyle, and personal preferences. The number of grams of Net Carbs one person can consume and continue to slim down on can vary significantly from that of another person. You might max out at 35 grams a day but your spouse may be able to continue to lose weight at 65 grams. An active eighteen-year-old woman is likely to metabolize carbohydrates much more rapidly than her menopausal mom.

To customize Atkins to your needs and preferences, you can:

- Stay in Phase 1 longer than two weeks if you have lots of weight to lose.
- Start in Phase 2 if you've just a few pounds to lose.

- Stay at the same carb intake for several weeks in Phases 2 and 3 instead of moving up after one or two weeks.
- Introduce new food categories more slowly instead of every week or two.
- Start in Phase 2 if you're willing to trade slower weight loss for more culinary variety.
- Change the order in which you reintroduce certain foods in a phase. For example, if you really miss berries, add them back before reintroducing nuts and seeds.
- Likewise, move to Phase 3 before you're 10 pounds from your goal weight if boredom with food choices could derail you.

Or you can even start in Phase 3 if you are content to lose weight considerably more slowly.

Also, remember you can do Atkins as a vegetarian, or even a vegan. Most vegetarians begin in Phase 2 so they can incorporate nuts and small portions of legumes immediately. A vegan would probably need to start in Phase 3 so he or she could include higher protein grains such as quinoa from the get-go. For more detail on how to customize Atkins to your needs, review Chapter 6 of *The New Atkins for a New You*.

WHAT CAN I EAT?

If you assume that losing weight means a limited number of choices and tasteless meals, you're in for a pleasant surprise. There are literally hundreds of foods you can eat from Day 1 on the new Atkins Diet. And since you can cook and dress your salads with natural oils, top veggies with butter, and enjoy a host of seasonings and condiments, you'll find Atkins cuisine deliciously flavorful. Fish, poultry, meat, and vegetarian protein choices such as tofu, as well as that perfect food, the egg, are on the menu from the start. You can also enjoy hard or aged cheese in moderation, and fresh cheeses and other dairy products such as Greek yogurt join the menu in Phase 2. Then there's also the vast world of vegetables. What we call "foundation vegetables" contain most of the carbs you'll consume in the early weeks of the program.

WHAT ARE FOUNDATION VEGETABLES?

The veggies you'll be eating from Day 1 include the leafy greens that are the foundation of salads—think arugula, lettuce in all its wondrous varieties, endive, radicchio—plus avocado, radishes, tomatoes, cucumbers, bean sprouts, celery, and scallions, for starters. Other foundation veggies, such as artichoke, spinach, chard, kale, cauliflower and its cruciferous cousins, plus green beans and zucchini—to name but a few—are usually cooked. Basically, any vegetable that's low in carbs—meaning the vast majority of them—is yours to savor from Phase 1 on. As a bonus, these carb misers are high in fiber as well as antioxidants and have plenty of other micronutrients.

That great diversity of flavors and textures available in foundation vegetables makes it easier to wait until Phase 3 to reintroduce the starchy, higher carb veggies, including winter squash, corn, and peas, and most root vegetables such as white potato and sweet potato. At that time you can also have grains and a wider array of fruits, although you may need to keep portions small unless you have a particularly high tolerance for carbs. For a list of some of the foods you'll be eating—and when you can eat them—see "What You Can Eat When" on page 21.

CONVENIENCE IS KEY

Atkins has always been primarily a whole-foods diet, but does that mean you have to be a chef or spend hours in the kitchen preparing low-carb meals and snacks from scratch? No way! We understand that your busy lifestyle means it often can be difficult to find the time to plan, shop, prepare, and store everything you eat. The good news is you can still do Atkins—and do it effortlessly. That's why Atkins Nutritionals provides "no-brainer" solutions for quick and easy meals and snacks with specially formulated and convenient low-carb products. In fact, these foods play a key role for most people on the program. When you're too busy to cook, are on the run, need a fast snack to tame the midafternoon munchies, or simply want to treat yourself to a low-carb dessert, these products are lifesavers.

Some Advantage bars are formulated to serve as an occasional meal replacement; others serve as snacks or can be paired with a protein source as a stand-in for a meal. A Day Break bar plus an Atkins shake make a great breakfast—or have the shake as a stand-alone snack. The Endulge line treats are a low-carb alternative to sky-high–carb candy bars. But wait, it gets better. Akins has recently introduced a line of frozen entrées that are not only delicious but have been designed to fit into all four phases of the diet. Made with fine ingredients such as freshly picked vegetables, sauces with real cream, and premium chicken, these meals are suitable for breakfast, lunch, and dinner. So you can stay on track—even when your schedule is packed or you're on the go. Check out the Atkins products in the Carb Counter, beginning on page 322. For more detail on product lines, carb counts, and the phases for which each product is suitable, go to www.atkins.com/Products.

PHASE 1 GUIDELINES

Poultry, fish, meat, eggs. Eat enough to satisfy but not stuff yourself. Have 4–6 ounces of protein foods at each meal, or up to 8 ounces if you're a big guy. There's no need to trim fat from meat or remove skin from poultry—but if you do, simply add a little olive oil or butter to your vegetables to replace the fat. Both dark and light meat are fine. Check the Net Carb counts on vegetarian protein products, which can vary dramatically. Roast, broil, grill, bake, stew, poach, sauté, or stir-fry but don't bread or batter-fry these foods. Cook eggs in any and every way you enjoy them. Just to be clear, Atkins is not a high-protein diet. Most people consume somewhere between 13 and 22 ounces of protein foods each day, making it more properly an optimal protein diet.

Cheese. Up to 4 ounces—each thin slice or 1¼-inch cube is roughly an ounce—of hard or aged cheese per day.

Foundation vegetables. To achieve the recommended minimum of 12–15 daily grams of Net Carbs have roughly six cups of salad veggies (each cup equals a serving, but you can certainly have more than one serving at a meal) and about two cups of cooked vegetables (½ cup is a typical serving). You can steam, stir-fry, sauté, braise, grill, or simmer veggies in soups. But never boil them, which destroys nutrients. The vegetables you select will determine the actual carb count and therefore the number of servings. Dress salads with oil and vinegar or lemon or lime juice or use prepared dressings with no more than 3 grams of Net Carbs per serving (1–2 table-spoons) and no added sugar.

Fats and oils. Regard a serving as 1 tablespoon, or a pat, of butter. If possible, opt for cold-pressed or expeller-pressed oils, which haven't been heated, leaving the nutrients intact. Extra-virgin olive oil is preferable for salads and dressing vegetables, but for cooking use olive, canola, high-oleic safflower, coconut, or grape-seed oil. Drizzle specialty oils such as walnut, sesame, flaxseed, or macadamia nut oil on food rather than heating them. When cooking food, use just enough oil to prevent the food from burning but not so much oil that the item swims in it.

Non-caloric sweeteners. Count each packet as 1 gram of Net Carbs and consume no more than three packets' worth a day. Although the sweeteners contain no carbs, the filler used with them does.

Condiments, herbs, and spices. Read labels to ferret out products with added sugars, flour, or cornstarch.

Beverages. Have no more than 3 tablespoons (1.5 ounces) a day of cream, and tally the carbs. You can count up to 2 cups of coffee or tea toward your water intake.

Low-carb foods. You can also enjoy Atkins bars, shakes, and frozen foods. (See "Convenience Is Key," and the Carb Counter on pages 298–324.)

HAVE THIS INSTEAD OF THAT

For most people, Induction is a relatively short period in which to jump-start weight loss and turn your body into a fat-burning machine. Instead of feeling deprived of foods you must temporarily forego, focus on the multitude of good foods you *can* eat. Besides, with the exception of "junk food," you'll be able to reintroduce most other foods as you move through the other phases. Substitutes for foods you'll put aside for now—or in some cases, for good—follow.

NO-NO	YES-YES
Fruit juice	Club soda or seltzer with a spritz of lemon or lime juice; bottled water flavored water with fruit essences; also Crystal Lite
Fruit	In Phase 1, rhubarb, which is technically a vegetable; sugar-free fruit gelatin desserts; berries in Phase 3; other fruits in Phase 3 and 4
Milk	Cream diluted with water; plain, unflavored soymilk, almond milk, coconut "dairy" beverage; reintroduce small amounts of milk in Phase 2
Colas and other soda	Calorie-free sodas, preferably sweetened with Splenda or stevia
Bread, pasta, tortillas, muffins, pastries, cookies, and chips	Low-carb specialty foods such as Atkins Day Break bars with no more than 3 grams of Net Carbs per serving; whole-grain products in Phase 3
Sugar, honey, etc.	Stevia, sucralose (stevia), saccharin, and xylitol
Candy	Atkins Endulge bars
Cookies and other sweet snacks	Low-carb specialty foods such as Atkins Advantage bars and shakes with no more than 3 grams of Net Carbs
Nuts and seeds and their butters	Flaxseeds; others are acceptable after 2 weeks in Induction
Low-fat foods	Conventional full-fat foods (check carb counts)
"Diet" or "low-fat" products	Atkins bars, shakes, and frozen entrées
Chewing gum and breath mints	Gum and mints sweetened with xylitol, sorbitol, or another sugar alcohol (up to 3 a day)
Cough syrup with added sugars	Sugar-free alternatives
Any food made with manufactured trans fats (hydrogenated or partially hydrogenated oils)	Trans-fat–free alternatives

WHAT AND WHERE ARE ADDED SUGARS?

The naturally occurring sugars in whole foods are integral to the food, which isn't to say you can eat them freely. Witness lactose, the sugar in milk, and fructose, the sugar in fruit, both of which you'll generally avoid in the earlier phases of Atkins. Then there are added sugars, which boost the sweetness of foods. They can be natural, such as the honey or maple syrup you may find in salad dressings or breakfast cereals, or manufactured, such as the high-fructose corn syrup found in most sodas. But natural or manu-factured, added sugars add up when it comes to your carb intake and your waistline. The good news is that according to a study published in 2011 in the *American Journal of Clinical Nutrition*, Americans are consuming 25 percent less added sugar than they did almost a decade ago. The decrease appears to be due to reduced consumption of sweetened beverages. However, it means that each person is still consuming an average of 306 calories per day as added sugar (compared to 400 calories earlier), more than 14 per-cent of typical daily calorie intake.

In addition to table sugar, brown sugar, raw sugar, and invert sugar, be on guard for the other names under which added sugar lurks. Check ingredient lists on packaged food for corn sweetener, corn syrup, corn syrup solids, dextrose, fructose, fruit juice concen-trate of any sort, glucose, high-fructose corn syrup, honey, lactose, maltose, malt, malt syrup, molasses, and sucrose.

CLIMBING THE CARB LADDER

The carb ladder prioritizes the order in which we recommend you reintroduce carbohydrate foods. The foods on the first two rungs are integral to Phase 1. Rungs 3–7 are usually reintroduced in Phase 2, and the remaining three rungs in Phase 3. All Atkins frozen entrées and shakes and most bars are suitable for Induction. Check labels for phase designations. Alcohol is not listed because it is not a food, but can be introduced in moderation and with certain exceptions in Phase 2. Finally, small amounts of dark chocolate without added sugar—including baking chocolate—are acceptable in Phase 2. Keep in mind that the higher a food is on the ladder, the more carbs it contains and therefore the less frequently you're likely to consume it.

PHASE	RUNG	FOOD	COMMENTS
1	1	Foundation vegetables	Leafy greens and other low-carb vegetables
1	2	Cream, sour cream, and most hard cheeses	Dairy foods high in fat and low in carbs
2	3	Nuts, seeds, and their butters	May be added after two weeks in Phase 1
2	4	Berries, cherries, and most melons	Excludes watermelon
2	5	Fresh cheeses like ricotta and cottage, whole milk yogurt	Plain unsweetened yogurt only
2	6	Legumes such as lentils, chickpeas, edamame	May postpone introduction to Phase 3
2	7	Tomato juice and tomato juice cocktail	Also more lemon or lime juice
3	8	Other fruits	But no fruit juice, dried fruits, or canned or frozen fruit with added sugar or syrup
3	9	Other vegetables	Starchy vegetables such as sweet potatoes, peas, sweet corn, carrots, and winter squash
3	10	Whole grains	Avoid refined grains such as white flour and products made with it

*You can also have small amounts of lemon or lime juice in Phase 1.

AVOID WEAKNESS AND FATIGUE WHEN YOU START ATKINS

When your body begins the process of converting to a primarily fat-burning metabolism, you may experience certain symptoms, which can include headaches, dizziness, weakness, and fatigue, as well as constipation. How come? Consuming carbs provokes an insulin spike that makes you retain water, which is why the first thing most people notice after a few days on Atkins is that they no longer feel bloated. This release of excess fluid can also lower your blood pressure, which is a good thing if you have hypertension. (If you take diuretics for this condition, talk to your doctor if your blood pressure drops naturally, as you may need to adjust your dosage.)

But when you excrete fluids, you also lose some electrolytes, such as sodium, which can account for dizziness, weakness, and, if you become dehydrated, constipation. The solution is to drink enough water and other clear fluids and to replace the lost sodium with a daily ½ teaspoon of salt. If you wish, you can instead have two cups of regular (not low-sodium) chicken, beef, or vegetable broth or 2 tablespoons of regular (not low-sodium) soy sauce sprinkled on your food over the day. Just to be clear, this doesn't make Atkins a high-sodium diet. All you're doing is rebalancing your electrolytes. I recommend you use this protocol when you start doing Atkins, rather than waiting to experience symptoms, which could interfere with your commitment to the program. After four weeks, your system should have adjusted to the metabolic change and then you can probably eliminate the extra sodium, although many people find having a cup of broth in the morning and another one in the afternoon to be a filling and comforting ritual.

WHEN YOU LEAVE PHASE 1

When you move on to Phase 2, slowly add back carbohydrate foods in the order listed in Climbing the Carb Ladder, allowing at least a week between categories such as nuts and seeds and berries, as long as you continue to lose weight. Also add only one type of food—sample walnuts, for example, before adding almonds—at a time so you can identify any food intolerances to see whether one food causes cravings or other reactions. Meanwhile, you'll also be increasing your overall carb intake incrementally—by 5 grams every week or several weeks. You can begin to consume some alcoholic beverages in moderation (see page 315 of the Carb Counter) and low-carb convenience foods with Net Carb counts of up to 6 grams.

As you approach your goal weight and move to Pre-Maintenance, you'll most likely be able to add back moderate amounts of the remaining carb foods in the order listed in Climbing the Carb Ladder. As you did in Phase 2, introduce one category at a time, as long as you continue to gradually lose weight, allowing a week or more between categories. Also continue to reintroduce only one type of fruit, starchy vegetable, or whole grain at a time to gauge any reaction. (If you didn't reintroduce legumes in Ongoing Weight Loss, OWL, you can do so now.) At the same time, try to increase your overall carb intake by 10 grams weekly or every few weeks until weight loss plateaus or you regain a pound or two. You can also begin to use low-carb food products with a Net Carb count of 7–9 grams. Stay in Phase 3 until you've reached and then maintained your goal weight for four weeks, before moving officially to Lifetime Maintenance.

THE PHASES DECODED

PHASE	1: INDUCTION	2: ONGOING WEIGHT LOSS	3. PRE-MAINTENANCE	4. LIFETIME MAINTENANCE
Objective	Train your body to burn primarily fat to jump-start weight loss.	Lose most of your excess weight as you reintroduce more foods and discover how many carbs you can consume while continuing to slim down.	Transition from weight loss to weight maintenance as you find the carb-intake level that lets you maintain your weight.	Fine-tune your carb tolerance and maintain your goal weight.
Duration	2 weeks or more	Variable	Variable	A lifetime
Daily Net Carbs	20 grams	25 grams or more	30 grams or more	30 grams or more
Start Here If You...	need to lose more than 30 pounds or want to take them off faster.	need to lose 15–30 pounds and are willing to do so more slowly than if you start in Phase 1.	have little or no weight to lose but want to improve your diet or health.	n/a

THE PHASES DECODED (*cont.*)

PHASE	1: INDUCTION	2: ONGOING WEIGHT LOSS	3. PRE-MAINTENANCE	4. LIFETIME MAINTENANCE
Acceptable Foods	Poultry, fish, meat, tofu, eggs, hard cheeses, "foundation vegetables," natural fats, condiments, suitable low-carb products, and sugar-free beverages	Rungs 3–7 of the Carb Ladder, plus more lemon and lime juice, some alcoholic beverages, suitable low-carb products, and sugar-free dark chocolate	Rungs 8–10 of the Carb Ladder	All whole foods if tolerated
Move to Next Phase	After 2 weeks or when you come within 15 pounds of goal weight, if you prefer	Usually at about 10 pounds from goal weight	Four weeks after you reach your goal weight	n/a
Comments	After two weeks add back nuts and seeds. Can stay here for months but it is important to move through the phases in order to segue to a permanent way of eating.	Move up in 5-gram daily increments each week or over several weeks as long as weight loss continues.	Move up in 10-gram daily increments each week or over several weeks as long as weight loss continues. Drop back 5 or 10 grams if weight loss stalls or reverses.	Make this your permanent way of eating.

WHAT YOU CAN EAT WHEN

	PHASE 1	PHASE 2	PHASE 3/4	AVOID
PROTEIN FOODS				
All fish	X	X	X	Batter-dipped or breaded fish, pickled herring with sugar
All shellfish				Artificial crab ("sea legs")
All poultry	X	X	X	Batter-dipped or breaded poultry and processed products
All meat	X	X	X	
Eggs	X	X	X	
Tofu, tofu "meat" and "cheese" analogs, seitan, and tempeh	X	X	X	
Veggie burger, crumbles and "meatballs"	X	X	X	Products with soy or other beans are not suitable for Phase 1
DAIRY PRODUCTS				
Aged or hard cheeses	X	X	X	Cheese spreads with fruit, "diet" cheese, "cheese products," and whey cheese
Cream cheese and other fresh cheeses, Greek yogurt (whole milk, plain)		X	X	Skim-milk or low-fat products
Cream and half-and-half	X	X	X	
Milk		X	X	Skim-milk or low-fat milk
VEGETABLES				
Avocado, Hass	X	X	X	Shiny green Florida avocados
Artichokes	X	X	X	
Asparagus	X	X	X	
Bamboo shoots	X	X	X	
Beets		X		
Bitter greens	X	X	X	
Beans, green and yellow	X	X	X	
Bean sprouts	X	X	X	
Bok choy and other Asian greens	X	X	X	
Lettuce, all kinds	X	X	X	

WHAT YOU CAN EAT WHEN (*cont.*)

	PHASE 1	PHASE 2	PHASE 3/4	AVOID
Broccoli, Brussels sprouts, cauliflower, etc.	X	X	X	
Cabbage and sauerkraut	X	X	X	
Carrots			X	
Cassava (yuca) and other tropical roots			X	
Celery and celery root (celeriac)	X	X	X	
Onions	X	X	X	
Corn			X	
Cucumber	X	X	X	
Radish and daikon	X	X	X	
Eggplant	X	X	X	
Fennel	X	X	X	
Jicama	X	X	X	
Kale	X	X	X	
Mushrooms	X	X	X	
Olives, black and green	X	X	X	
Palm, hearts of	X	X	X	
Parsley and other fresh herbs	X	X	X	
Parsnips, rutabaga, Jerusalem artichoke			X	
Peas			X	
Peppers, bell and chili	X	X	X	
Potatoes (white), sweet potatoes, and yams			X	
Pumpkin	X	X	X	
Radish and daikon	X	X	X	
Rhubarb, unsweetened	X	X	X	
Snow peas, snap peas in the pod	X	X	X	

WHAT YOU CAN EAT WHEN (*cont.*)

	PHASE 1	PHASE 2	PHASE 3/4	AVOID
Spaghetti squash	X	X	X	
Spinach and Swiss chard	X	X	X	
Tomato and tomatillo	X	X	X	
Water chestnuts	X	X	X	
Winter squash		X		
Zucchini and other summer squash	X	X	X	
FATS, OILS, AND SALAD DRESSINGS				
Butter	X	X	X	
Cooking oil	X	X	X	Soybean, sunflower, "regular" safflower, corn, or "vegetable" oil
Nut and seed oils	X	X	X	Peanut oil
Mayonnaise (made with olive, canola, or high-oleic safflower oil)				Products with soybean oil or added sugar; low-fat products
Salad dressings (vinaigrette, blue cheese, Caesar, Italian, ranch)	X	X	X	Prepared dressings made with sugar; low-fat products
SWEETENERS				
Sucralose (Splenda)	X	X	X	
Stevia (Truvia, SweetLeaf, etc.)	X	X	X	
Saccharin (Sweet 'N Low)	X	X	X	
Xylitol	X	X	X	
CONDIMENTS, HERBS, AND SPICES				
Anchovy paste	X	X	X	
Black bean sauce	X	X	X	
Capers	X	X	X	
Chili powder, chipotle en adobo	X	X	X	
Coconut milk, unsweetened	X	X	X	

WHAT YOU CAN EAT WHEN (*cont.*)

	PHASE 1	PHASE 2	PHASE 3/4	AVOID
Cocoa powder, unsweetened	X	X	X	
Enchilada, taco, sauce	X	X	X	
Fish sauce	X	X	X	
Garlic	X	X	X	
Ginger	X	X	X	
Horseradish sauce	X	X	X	
Miso paste	X	X	X	
Mustard	X	X	X	Honey mustard or others with added sugar
Pesto sauce	X	X	X	
Pickle, dill or Kosher	X	X	X	Sweet pickles
Pimento (roasted red pepper)	X	X	X	
Salsa, green or red	X	X	X	Products with added sugar
Soy sauce and tamari	X	X	X	
Spices, dried herbs, curry powder, and other spice mixtures	X	X	X	Spice blends made with sugar
Tabasco or other hot sauce	X	X	X	
Vinegar	X	X	X	Rice vinegar with sugar
Wasabi paste	X	X	X	
BEVERAGES				
Clear broth/bouillon	X	X	X	Low-sodium products or ones with added sugar
Club soda	X	X	X	
Caffeinated or decaf coffee	X	X	X	
Caffeinated or decaf tea and herb tea	X	X	X	

THE NEW ATKINS FOR A NEW YOU WORKBOOK

WHAT YOU CAN EAT WHEN (*cont.*)

	PHASE 1	PHASE 2	PHASE 3/4	AVOID
Diet sodas sweetened with noncaloric sweeteners	X	X	X	
Lemon or lime juice	X	X	X	
Seltzer, plain or essence flavored	X	X	X	
Soy, almond, or coconut "dairy" beverages	X	X	X	Products with added sugars
Sugar-free mixers	X	X	X	
Tomato juice or vegetable juice "cocktail"		X	X	
Water, tap, spring, filtered, or mineral	X	X	X	
ALCOHOLIC BEVERAGES	Sugary wine coolers, cordials, or any beverage with a high sugar content			
Beer, "lite" or low carb		X	X	
Champagne		X	X	
Gin, vodka, or white rum		X	X	
Sherry, dry		X	X	Sweet sherry
Spirits, white or brown		X	X	
Wine, red, white, rosé, dry white dessert		X	X	
NUTS AND SEEDS				
All tree nuts		X	X	Chestnuts
Coconut, unsweetened		X	X	Products with added sugars
Peanuts		X	X	
Nut and seed butters (including tahini)		X	X	Products with added sugars
Soy "nuts" and "nut" butter		X	X	
BERRIES AND FRUITS				
Apples		X		
Banana and plantain		X		
Berries, all kinds		X	X	Frozen berries should contain no added sugar

WHAT YOU CAN EAT WHEN (*cont.*)

	PHASE 1	PHASE 2	PHASE 3/4	AVOID
Cherries, sour and sweet		X	X	Frozen cherries should contain no added sugar
Figs			X	
Melon (except watermelon)		X	X	
Grapes			X	
Guava			X	
Kiwifruit			X	
Lychee			X	
Mango, papaya, and other tropical fruits			X	
Oranges, grapefruit, and other citrus fruits		X		
Peaches, plums, and other stone fruits			X	
Pears			X	
Persimmon			X	
Pineapple			X	
Pomegranate			X	
Quince			X	
Watermelon			X	
LEGUMES				
Lentils, chickpeas, and all legumes		X	X	Baked beans made with sugar
Bean dips		X	X	Products with added starches or sugars
WHOLE GRAINS				
Bran, wheat or oat	X	X	X	
Corn meal and hominy			X	
Oatmeal, steel cut or rolled			X	Products with added sugar
Rice, bulgur, and other whole grains			X	
100 percent whole-grain breads and other baked goods			X	Products with added sugar and/or white flour

THE NEW ATKINS FOR A NEW YOU WORKBOOK

	PHASE 1	PHASE 2	PHASE 3/4	AVOID
ATKINS PRODUCTS				
Atkins Advantage bars and shakes*	X	X	X	
Atkins Day Break bars	X	X	X	
Atkins Endulge bars*	X	X	X	
Atkins frozen entrées	X	X	X	

*A few bars are not coded for Phase 1. Check the package for phase designation. For Net Carb counts for these and other foods, see the Carb Counter at the end of this workbook. For a more complete carb counter, go to www.atkins.com/tools.

HOW DO I PUT TOGETHER MEALS?

Now that you have a good idea of the variety of foods you can eat on Atkins, even in Phase 1, how do you actually set up your menus? Base your meals around your preferred protein sources, natural fats, and foundation vegetables. Plan on three meals and one or two snacks a day, or five small meals if that works better for you. Veggies should comprise the majority of your carb intake. Cheese, cream for your coffee or tea, eggs—a large egg contains 0.4 grams of Net Carbs—lemon juice, vinegar, and other condiments will bring your tally up to 20 grams a day. If you use acceptable noncaloric sweeteners (sucralose [Spenda], stevia [Truvia or SweetLeaf], saccharin [Sweet'N Low], or xylitol), count 1 gram of Net Carbs per packet— the sweeteners themselves are carb free, but the packets use filler that contains carbs. It's best to spread your carb intake across the day.

If you exceed your intake by a couple of grams one day, simply cut back the next day, as long as you don't exceed 22 grams or go lower than 18 grams. Eating too many carbs could stall your fat-burning engine; eating too few almost certainly means you won't be getting enough foundation vegetables full of vitamins, minerals, fiber, and other good things. Feel free to use phase-appropriate Atkins products in moderation but not at the expense of foundation veggies.

In Phase 1, a typical day might look like this:

- Breakfast: two eggs in any style with a few tomato slices and a sausage patty, plus coffee or tea with cream
- *Midmorning snack:* cucumber hollowed out and smeared with cream cheese, or an Atkins Day Break bar
- *Lunch:* Cobb salad topped with grilled chicken and tossed with blue cheese dressing or an Atkins frozen entrée such as Crustless Chicken Pot Pie
- *Afternoon snack:* an Atkins Advantage shake
- *Dinner:* grilled salmon drizzled with lemon juice, a salad with avocado and tossed with vinaigrette, and sautéed zucchini

Assuming proper portion sizes, this meal plan would come in at roughly 20 grams of Net Carbs, of which 12–15 would come from foundation vegetables (the tomato, cucumber, two salads, avocado, and zucchini). The eggs, sausage, chicken, and salmon would provide sufficient protein. Note that carb foods should always be consumed with protein or fat to blunt the impact on your blood sugar. Rather than have a "naked" cucumber as a snack, for example, have it with cheese (or in later phases with some nuts). Ditto for any other vegetable. On the other hand, you could have cheese or nuts (after the first two weeks of Induction) alone, if you wish, as a snack—they contain both carbs and fats, as well as some protein.

DON'T OVERDO THE FAT

Although Atkins encourages you to enjoy the natural fats and oils that you'll be burning for energy, along with your excess body fat, there can be too much of a good thing. After all, fat is more than twice as dense in calories as protein and carbohydrate. In a typical day, plan on having the following: a couple of tablespoons of olive or other oils for salad dressings and cooking, a tablespoon of butter on cooked veggies, an ounce of cream in coffee or tea, a couple of ounces of cheese, two or three eggs, and the same number of servings of meat, poultry, or seafood, ten olives, half a Hass avocado, and 2 ounces of nuts or seeds (after the first two weeks of Phase 1). Some people may have a bit more, others a bit less, depending upon their height and build. You'll find the right amount for you, based upon your weight-loss progress.

HOW ABOUT BREAKFAST?

If you've been used to having cold cereal, breakfast pastries, or toast for breakfast, you need to rethink your options. Eggs, of course, are always on the menu. Other Phase 1 breakfast suggestions include these:

- sautéed ground beef with vegetables
- an Atkins Advantage shake plus some added protein, such as a slice of cheese
- sliced turkey or ham rolled around cheese and steamed veggies
- An Atkins frozen breakfast entrée
- smoked salmon rolled around cream cheese and sliced cucumber
- Mashed cauliflower topped with Cheddar cheese and bacon
- an Atkins Day Break bar with a hard boiled egg
- last night's leftovers reheated

AND HOW ABOUT SNACKS?

In addition to Atkins Advantage and Day Break shakes and bars, other Induction snack suggestions include these:

- a hard-boiled or deviled egg
- half an avocado
- celery stalk filled with blue cheese
- radishes with Cheddar cheese
- black or green olives
- marinated artichoke hearts
- string cheese
- roasted red peppers with goat cheese

For two weeks of Phase 1 meal plans, go to www.atkins.com/AtkinsDotCom/media/Master/Free%20Tools/Induction-Made-Easy-Final.pdf. To customize meal plans to your phase, Net Carb intake, and culinary preferences, become a member of the Atkins Community at community.atkins.com.

OTHER TIPS FOR SUCCESS

PROPER PORTIONS ARE KEY TO SUCCESS

Knowing what you can eat in each phase of Atkins is essential to achieving your goals, but equally important is to understand and practice portion control. Obviously, if you eat too much of any food, whether parsley or pork chops, you could simply consume so much food that your body's fat stores are never tapped. But without knowing how much mashed cauliflower—a great substitute for mashed potato, by the way—you ate at dinner, you cannot calculate the number of grams of Net Carbs you consumed. And without knowing that, your goose is cooked, so to speak. Until you know the number of grams of carbs you can eat to lose weight (and later maintain weight), you're playing carb roulette, hoping you're betting on the right number with no realistic idea if you are.

Fortunately, you don't have to actually go through the tedious and boring process of measuring food in tablespoons and cups to track your carb intake. Instead, start out using some familiar visuals and, quickly, you'll be able to estimate a 4- or 6-ounce portion of meat or fish, or a half-cup portion of steamed spinach or braised zucchini.

FOOD	VISUAL
4 ounces meat, poultry, fish, tofu, etc.	A large matchbox
6 ounces meat, poultry, fish, tofu, etc.	A hockey puck
8 ounces meat, poultry, tofu, etc.	A slim paperback book
1 ounce hard cheese	Four dice
1 cup salad greens	A baseball or a small hand holding a tennis ball
½ cup cooked vegetables or grains	A lightbulb or a racquet or billiard ball
¼ cup cooked legumes	An egg
2 tablespoons nut butter	A golf ball or two Ping-Pong balls
½ cup cooked grains	A tennis ball

Alternatively, measure foods the first few times you have them, and you'll be able to eyeball portions going forward.

THE ROLE OF EXERCISE IN WEIGHT CONTROL

Do you need to exercise to lose weight on Atkins? No—and yes. You can definitely shed pounds without lifting a finger other than to reach your mouth, and if you're a long-term couch potato, you may want to get comfortable with the Atkins Diet before adding a fitness regimen to your new lifestyle. There's actually no evidence that exercising helps *everyone* lose weight—our genes appear to play a large role here—although there *is* convincing evidence that regular exercise allows people to maintain a healthy weight. That said, doing Atkins and engaging in regular physical activity is an ideal combination and offers excellent physical as well as mental health benefits. Cutting carbs will allow you to lose your excess body fat, but only exercise will tone your body by building muscle. Contrary to popular opinion, your fat does not magically morph into muscle. The loss of body fat and the building of muscle are two separate examples of cause and effect. But exercise does work hand in glove with a low-carb diet to unlock your fat stores.

The many other benefits of exercise include:

- enhanced energy
- improved mood
- reduced stress
- a sense of accomplishment
- preservation of lean body mass
- cardiovascular support
- better circulation
- reduced risk of degenerative diseases such as arthritis

THE IMPORTANCE OF SETTING GOALS

Without specific goals, it can be difficult to stick to a plan of action and all too easy to put off until tomorrow what you'd rather not do today. Only problem is when tomorrow rolls around, you're still not in the mood, and before long your desire to change things in your life is just that: an unfulfilled wish. On the other hand, establishing goals allows you to gauge the distance between where you are now and where you want to be and to plot your course to get from Point A to Point B. Motivating yourself can be hard at times, but when your goals are down in black and white, there's no question that it's easier to stick to your guns.

CHANGE BEGETS CHANGE

By purchasing this workbook, you've declared your intention to make significant changes in how you eat and how you look and feel. It may be scary but you've decided to go ahead and move into un-charted territory that will give you a new way of looking at yourself. Somewhere along the line, what used to be an effort—whether eating properly, taking regular brisk walks, or eliminating sugary beverages—becomes the only path you can envision. You've created a whole new set of habits.

As you begin to effect changes—in your self-control, your shrinking waistline, perhaps even your attitude toward exercise— you'll feel empowered not just by the positive changes themselves but by your resolve to achieve them. Over and over again, I've seen

THE NEW ATKINS FOR A NEW YOU WORKBOOK

people who take control of their weight and therefore their health begin to make other life changes, whether it's changing careers, beginning or ending a relationship, returning to college, or volunteering to help others in one way or another.

TEN UNBREAKABLE RULES

To maximize your results on the new Atkins Diet—head off binges—follow these rules:

1. Track your daily carb intake.
2. Eat only foods listed above.
3. Don't skip meals.
4. Don't "starve" yourself or go more than six waking hours without eating.
5. Don't restrict fats.
6. Learn the difference between hunger and habit: Eat only until you're satisfied, not stuffed. When in doubt, wait ten minutes, drink a glass of water, and have more food only if you're still unsatisfied.
7. Before eating any packaged food, read the ingredients lists on food labels to check the grams of Net Carbs and see if it contains added sugars.
8. Stick with Atkins low-carb products, which have verified minimal impact on blood sugar.
9. Drink a minimum of eight daily 8-ounce glasses of water and other acceptable beverages (or enough to keep your urine clear or pale yellow). By doing so, you'll flush toxins from your system and enhance your body's ability to metabolize fat for energy.
10. Take a daily multivitamin/mineral and an omega-3 supplement.

Be sure to set realistic goals. Particularly if you have a large number of pounds to shed, you may find it more motivating to set a series of incremental goals. For example, in the first two months, aim to lose 20 pounds and then another 5 pounds each month after that. You can do the same with fitness. Start taking a one-mile walk three times a week and gradually reset your time and frequency as you build your endurance.

HOW TO USE THIS WORKBOOK

Congratulations on your decision to make big changes that will impact your appearance, health, and self-confidence for years to come. This workbook will help you set your goals and then stay on top of them. It will also serve as a gentle reminder of the reasons you decided to do Atkins in the first place and the forces that motivate you to stick with the program. Each week you'll strategize the week ahead, as well as log in the numbers that represent your progress. You'll also have an opportunity to reflect on the changes in your body—and in your life.

The journal contains two types of pages:

Week by week. Before you begin, you'll have the opportunity to enter your benchmark ("before") numbers for your weight, key measurements, BMI, and WHR (waist-to-hip ratio), as well as write about your emotions, reasons for deciding to embark on the new Atkins Diet, and other such matters. From the end of Week 1 on, you'll have a place to take stock of where you are, including your weight and measurements, plus plenty of space to note the challenges you're facing, the solutions you're coming up with, and your thoughts and feelings about the process. (Note that you'll weigh and measure yourself only once a week to avoid obsessing about meaningless day-to-day changes in your weight.) These pages also provide a set of questions to help you decide whether to move from one phase to the next or to reintroduce a new food category as you plan for the week to come.

LEARN THE LAW OF AVERAGES

Although I recommend you weigh and measure yourself only once a week, if you have a serious attachment to your scale, a less obsessive approach is to average your weight daily. This is a better indicator or your progress (or what you could perceive as a failure to progress) than a single day's weight. To do so, weigh yourself each day at the same time of day and record the number. The next day and the following one, do the same. Add those numbers together and divide them by three to average your weight. Continue to keep a running tally. It is unreasonable to expect to lose weight every day–and a number of body processes will influence your weight throughout the day and even from day to day.

Day by day. On these pages you'll record everything you eat and drink, along with serving size and Net Carb counts, using the Carb Counter on page 298, and tally the daily total to see whether you're staying on track. For simplicity's sake, only Net Carbs are provided, as they're the only ones you have to count on Atkins. (The fiber in vegetables, grains, legumes, berries, fruit, and other foods gets a free ride, as it passes through your GI tract without impacting your blood sugar.) For optimal success in keeping your journal:

- Tell the whole truth. Be sure to enter everything you consume, including condiments and toppings, even if it's a food that you'd be better off avoiding.
- Precision counts. Indicate your portion sizes and check out the nutritional information on packaged foods.
- Be consistent. Always carry this workbook with you so you don't have to rely on your recollections hours later. And just in case you occasionally forget, check out the new Atkins smartphone app that helps you track your intake at www.atkins.com.

Our memories often fail us, but keeping a written record will help you to see the cause and effect of eating or not eating certain foods. For example, if the progress you'd been making stalled after a close encounter with a Cinnabon, next time you encounter its seductive scent in the food court, you'll be better able to resist.

Here you can also list any physical activities, from workouts at a gym, to a yoga class, a walk, a jog, or whatever. Also note whether you've taken your vitamin/mineral and omega-3 supplements (See "Why Are Supplements Necessary?") and your daily intake of salt, soy sauce, or salty broth.

As in the weekly pages, you'll also have space to reflect upon your experiences.

WHY ARE SUPPLEMENTS NECESSARY?

If eating the Atkins way is nutritionally sound, why do you need anything else? Vitamins, minerals, antioxidants, and other micronutrients are vital to good health and your body's ability to function at peak performance. The Atkins Diet is nutrient rich, due to both the foundation veggies full of vitamins and minerals that comprise most of your initial carb intake and the protein and natural fats you'll be consuming. But all too often food travels great distances from field to supermarket, losing nutrients along the way. Also, in some locations soil may be depleted of nutrients, reducing the quality of vegetables and fruit. Cooking kills still more nutrients. The reality is that many Americans are deficient in several key micronutrients. As an insurance policy, we recommend you take the following:

- a daily multivitamin/mineral supplement that includes magnesium and calcium
- an omega-3 supplement (either fish oil or a plant substitute)
- an additional vitamin D supplement if you stay out of the sun, live in a northern climate, or use sunscreen routinely

A NOTE OF CLARIFICATION

As I've explained, the new Atkins Diet is extremely flexible, meaning you can personalize it to your needs. This very flexibility poses a bit of a challenge in this workbook. We can't assume that everyone will be in the same phase at the same time. Each week you'll indicate the phase you're in, as well as your target carb intake. However, you may have 20 pounds to banish and need to spend only two weeks in Induction before moving on to Ongoing Weight Loss, while your friend who is starting Atkins at the same time may have 35 pounds to pare off and expects to stay in Phase 1 for at least a month and likely longer. Assuming all things are equal, you'll be moving through the first three phases more rapidly than he or she will and you'll probably reach your goal weight before the sixteen weeks represented in this guide. Your friend may well take several more weeks or even months. All well and good, but the reason I mention this here is that the introductions to each week of the workbook often mention specific phases. That doesn't in any way suggest that you or anyone else should be in that phase at that time. I only attempt to address what you or any other reader may or may not experience as you move through the phases.

So, let's get going!

WEEK 1

Place your "before" photo here.

Me before I began
the new Atkins Diet.

Before you begin your weight-loss journey on the new Atkins Diet, you'll want to establish your baseline stats. Doing so will allow you to track your progress in pounds and inches lost and in positive shifts in your BMI and WHR indicators, as well as how you feel about your progress. Responding to the questions that follow will also help you understand your motivation and further strengthen your resolve to achieve your goals. Be as specific and truthful as possible. Remember, this workbook is for your eyes only. The payoff is that you'll see clear-cut evidence of your progress in the weeks to come.

Name: LUNA

Age: 29

Start date: 9-8-2013

MY CURRENT STATS

Chest: _____ inches   Waist: _____ inches

Hips: _____ inches   Upper arms: _____ inches

Thighs: _____ inches   Calves: _____ inches

Weight: 220 pounds   Dress Size/Pant Size: _____

BMI (see page 8) 41.56   WHR (see page 9) _____

Enter your current blood pressure and any other health statistics your physician may have provided you with. 120/84 , A1C 10.7 , fasting blood glucose 229

What made you decide to lose weight? miscarriage

Was there one pivotal event or occasion that made you decide to start now? If so, describe: I hate myself

What are your reasons for choosing the Atkins Diet? blood glucose / diabetes control

In which phase (see page 8) do you plan to start and how many daily grams of Net Carbs do you plan to consume? phase 1 20 NC

What is your goal weight and how long do you anticipate it will take you to reach it? 115 , 2 yrs

What are your other goals, such as fitness, health, and energy-enhancement ones and/or taking responsibility for your well-being?

NONE

If this is not the first time you've embarked on a weight-loss diet, briefly describe your previous experience(s) and what you learned from it/them that would inform your decisions now.

They work, I guess.

Are there any factors that might create challenges, such as frequent travel, business meals, family issues, or medications that interfere with weight loss? If so, how do you plan to deal with them?

Adjust insulin. Try to not give up when depression hits.

Do you currently eat a lot of snack foods, sweetened beverages, and sugary treats? Yes

Do you currently eat many vegetables? Yes

Are you hungry a few hours after a meal? Yes

Do you currently take a multivitamin, an omega-3 supplement, and/or a vitamin D supplement? Yes

Do you exercise never, rarely, occasionally, or regularly? Please describe: 3 times a week

Do you drink at least eight 8-ounce glasses of water and other clear fluids a day? _No_

Are your fridge, freezer, and pantry full of Atkins-friendly foods? _No_

How do imagine your life will change when you reach your goals?

I want a healthy baby

Are you ready to become the "new you"? _Yes_

Welcome to Week 1 on Atkins.

Date: 9-8-2013

TODAY'S MEALS (including portion sizes)

Breakfast: Grams Net Carbs

Subtotal: _____

Snack:

Lunch:

Subtotal: _____

Snack:

Dinner:

Subtotal: _____
Total grams Net Carbs: _____

Number of servings of foundation vegetables: _____
Did you take your multivitamin/mineral?   ❏ YES   ❏ NO
Your omega-3 supplement?   ❏ YES   ❏ NO
Your vitamin D supplement?   ❏ YES   ❏ NO
Did you have the recommended salt, soy sauce,
or broth?   ❏ YES   ❏ NO
Number of glasses of water: _____

TODAY'S JOURNAL

How are you doing on the diet? _____

_____

_____

How do you feel? _____

_____

_____

What's working for you? _____

_____

_____

Are you experiencing any challenges and how do you plan to overcome them? _____

_____

_____

How do you feel about the changes you're making? _____

_____

_____

Did you exercise today? _____
If so, what did you do and for how long? _____

_____

_____

_____

"The way to get started is to quit talking and begin doing."

—*Walt Disney*

Date: _____

TODAY'S MEALS (including portion sizes)

Breakfast: Grams Net Carbs

_____   _____
_____   _____
_____   _____

                              Subtotal: _____

Snack:

_____   _____

Lunch:

_____   _____
_____   _____
_____   _____
_____   _____

                              Subtotal: _____

Snack:

_____   _____

Dinner:

_____   _____
_____   _____
_____   _____
_____   _____

                              Subtotal: _____
                  Total grams Net Carbs: _____

Number of servings of foundation vegetables: _____
Did you take your multivitamin/mineral?   ❏ YES ❏ NO
Your omega-3 supplement?   ❏ YES ❏ NO
Your vitamin D supplement?   ❏ YES ❏ NO
Did you have the recommended salt, soy sauce,
or broth?   ❏ YES ❏ NO
Number of glasses of water: _____

TODAY'S JOURNAL

How are you doing on the diet? _____
_____

How do you feel? _____
_____

What's working for you? _____
_____

Are you experiencing any challenges and how do you plan to overcome them? _____
_____

How do you feel about the changes you're making? _____
_____

Did you exercise today? _____
If so, what did you do and for how long? _____
_____
_____

FOR A NEW YOU

GET PARTICULAR

The more specific (and realistic) your goals, the more likely you are to reach them. Instead of just declaring your desire to lose weight, be specific about how many pounds you plan to banish or the dress or waist size you plan to achieve. Also set a reasonable time frame within which to reach this goal. That's not to say that you can foretell the future, but specificity will help you avoid rationalizing why you can have that doughnut just this one time or swap out your foundation vegetables for a slice of pizza. Remember, you can always adjust your goals as you move forward.

Date: _____

TODAY'S MEALS (including portion sizes)

Breakfast: Grams Net Carbs
_____   _____
_____   _____
_____   _____

                              Subtotal: _____
Snack:
_____   _____
Lunch:
_____   _____
_____   _____
_____   _____
_____   _____

                              Subtotal: _____
Snack:
_____   _____
Dinner:
_____   _____
_____   _____
_____   _____
_____   _____

                              Subtotal: _____
                  Total grams Net Carbs: _____

Number of servings of foundation vegetables: _____
Did you take your multivitamin/mineral?   ❏ YES ❏ NO
Your omega-3 supplement?   ❏ YES ❏ NO
Your vitamin D supplement?   ❏ YES ❏ NO
Did you have the recommended salt, soy sauce,
or broth?   ❏ YES ❏ NO
Number of glasses of water: _____

TODAY'S JOURNAL

How are you doing on the diet? _____
_____

How do you feel? _____
_____

What's working for you? _____
_____

Are you experiencing any challenges and how do you plan to over-
come them? _____
_____

How do you feel about the changes you're making? _____
_____

Did you exercise today? _____
If so, what did you do and for how long? _____
_____
_____

RECENT RESEARCH

BELLY FAT CAN WEAKEN BONES

You probably know that carrying excess weight around your
middle increases your risk of heart disease, insulin resistance,
and type 2 diabetes. But only very thin women need to worry
about osteoporosis, right? Not so. Research at Massachusetts
General Hospital suggests that the fat that surrounds your or-
gans and pads your waist actually increases a woman's risk of
developing osteoporosis. Using high-tech methods, researchers looked at the bone marrow fat in a particular vertebra in
the spine of each study subject and then measured its bone-
mineral density. Women with more abdominal fat had lower
bone density, a sign of osteoporosis, but it was not associated
with the fat that lies directly under the skin.

Date: _____

TODAY'S MEALS (including portion sizes)

Breakfast: Grams Net Carbs

_____   _____

_____   _____

_____   _____

                              Subtotal: _____

Snack:

_____   _____

Lunch:

_____   _____

_____   _____

_____   _____

_____   _____

                              Subtotal: _____

Snack:

_____   _____

Dinner:

_____   _____

_____   _____

_____   _____

_____   _____

                              Subtotal: _____

                    Total grams Net Carbs: _____

Number of servings of foundation vegetables: _____

Did you take your multivitamin/mineral?   ❏ YES   ❏ NO

Your omega-3 supplement?   ❏ YES   ❏ NO

Your vitamin D supplement?   ❏ YES   ❏ NO

Did you have the recommended salt, soy sauce,
or broth?   ❏ YES   ❏ NO

Number of glasses of water: _____

TODAY'S JOURNAL

How are you doing on the diet? _____

_____

How do you feel? _____

_____

What's working for you? _____

_____

Are you experiencing any challenges and how do you plan to over-
come them? _____

_____

How do you feel about the changes you're making? _____

_____

Did you exercise today? _____
If so, what did you do and for how long? _____

_____

_____

REGULAR BENEFITS

Salad greens and other foundation vegetables contain lots of
fiber, which is why their carb counts are minimal. Consuming
that fiber, along with drinking enough fluids, will go a long
way toward avoiding constipation, which sometimes occurs
in the first few weeks after starting Atkins. Fiber also helps
stabilize your blood sugar and insulin levels, helping to keep
your appetite under control.

Date: _____

TODAY'S MEALS (including portion sizes)

Breakfast: Grams Net Carbs

_____   _____

_____   _____

_____   _____

                               Subtotal: _____

Snack:

_____   _____

Lunch:

_____   _____

_____   _____

_____   _____

_____   _____

                               Subtotal: _____

Snack:

_____   _____

Dinner:

_____   _____

_____   _____

_____   _____

_____   _____

                               Subtotal: _____

                    Total grams Net Carbs: _____

Number of servings of foundation vegetables: _____

Did you take your multivitamin/mineral?   ❏ YES   ❏ NO

Your omega-3 supplement?   ❏ YES   ❏ NO

Your vitamin D supplement?   ❏ YES   ❏ NO

Did you have the recommended salt, soy sauce,
or broth?   ❏ YES   ❏ NO

Number of glasses of water: _____

TODAY'S JOURNAL

How are you doing on the diet? _____

_____

_____

How do you feel? _____

_____

_____

What's working for you? _____

_____

_____

Are you experiencing any challenges and how do you plan to over-
come them? _____

_____

_____

How do you feel about the changes you're making? _____

_____

_____

Did you exercise today? _____
If so, what did you do and for how long? _____

_____

_____

_____

"You must act as if it is impossible to fail."

—*Ashanti Proverb*

Date: _____

TODAY'S MEALS (including portion sizes)

Breakfast: Grams Net Carbs

_____   _____

_____   _____

_____   _____

                               Subtotal: _____

Snack:

Lunch:

_____   _____

_____   _____

_____   _____

_____   _____

                               Subtotal: _____

Snack:

_____   _____

Dinner:

_____   _____

_____   _____

_____   _____

_____   _____

                               Subtotal: _____

                    Total grams Net Carbs: _____

Number of servings of foundation vegetables: _____

Did you take your multivitamin/mineral?   ❏ YES ❏ NO

Your omega-3 supplement?   ❏ YES ❏ NO

Your vitamin D supplement?   ❏ YES ❏ NO

Did you have the recommended salt, soy sauce,
or broth?   ❏ YES ❏ NO

Number of glasses of water: _____

TODAY'S JOURNAL

How are you doing on the diet? _____

_____

How do you feel? _____

_____

What's working for you? _____

_____

Are you experiencing any challenges and how do you plan to over-
come? _____

_____

How do you feel about the changes you're making? _____

_____

Did you exercise today? _____
If so, what did you do and for how long? _____

_____

_____

FOR A NEW YOU

ANOTHER REASON TO ENJOY OLIVE OIL

Olive oil has a delightfully complex flavor, but that's not the
only reason it's a good choice for your salads and cooked vegetables. One of the micronutrients in olives is oleocanthal,
which has robust anti-inflammatory properties. Increasingly,
inflammation is being linked to heart diseases, so eating anti-
inflammatory foods is part of the recipe for good health.

Date: _____

TODAY'S MEALS (including portion sizes)

Breakfast: Grams Net Carbs

_____   _____

_____   _____

_____   _____

                              Subtotal: _____

Snack:

_____   _____

Lunch:

_____   _____

_____   _____

_____   _____

_____   _____

                              Subtotal: _____

Snack:

_____   _____

Dinner:

_____   _____

_____   _____

_____   _____

_____   _____

                              Subtotal: _____

                   Total grams Net Carbs: _____

Number of servings of foundation vegetables: _____

Did you take your multivitamin/mineral?   ❏ YES ❏ NO

Your omega-3 supplement?   ❏ YES ❏ NO

Your vitamin D supplement?   ❏ YES ❏ NO

Did you have the recommended salt, soy sauce,
or broth?   ❏ YES ❏ NO

Number of glasses of water: _____

TODAY'S JOURNAL

How are you doing on the diet? _____

_____

How do you feel? _____

_____

What's working for you? _____

_____

Are you experiencing any challenges and how do you plan to over-
come them? _____

_____

Did you exercise today? _____
If so, what did you do and for how long? _____

_____

_____

RECENT RESEARCH

GOOD NEWS FOR YO-YO DIETERS

For years it was assumed that people who repeatedly lost
and regained weight made their metabolism less effective,
sabotaging future weight loss. Fortunately, a 2012 study published in *Metabolism* appears to contradict this assumption.
The study was based on data from 439 overweight or obese
older and sedentary women, some of whom were categorized
as either severe or moderate yo-yo dieters. The women were
randomly assigned to one of four groups: one that was put
on a weight-loss diet, one that required only exercise (mostly
brisk walking), one that combined diet and exercise, and one
that made neither change. After a year, the women in the diet
and the diet-exercise-combination groups averaged a 10 percent loss of their baseline weight. Although both groups of
yo-yo dieters were initially heavier than the other women,
there was no significant difference in their results compared
to those who had not yo-yoed in the past.

WEEK 2

Congratulations on completing your first week on Atkins! You're on your way to achieving your goals. Water weight disappears first, and by now you're probably beginning to shed some fat pounds, which initially come from your tummy. Some people lose a steady pound or half pound a day in the early weeks, but you may not experience weight loss for several days and then suddenly drop 2 or 3 pounds. That's why having set expectations in the short run could set you up for disappointment. It's also why I strongly recommend you steer clear of both the scale and the measuring tape until you've been doing Atkins for a week. Thereafter, continue to check your stats only once a week, weighing yourself at roughly the same time of day for the most valid comparison. (If you are hung up on the scale, review "Learn the Law of Averages" on page 35.) Be sure to measure at the same time you weigh in. Those numbers may decline before the pounds, making the way your clothes fit often the first sign of progress. Keep up your good work!

Phase: _____ Daily Net Carb Target: _____ grams

MY CURRENT STATS

Chest: _____ inches Waist: _____ inches
Hips: _____ inches Upper arms: _____ inches
Thighs: _____ inches Calves: _____ inches
Weight: _____ pounds
BMI: _____   WHR: _____

How do you feel about your results over the previous week? _____
_____
_____

Did you miss any particular foods? If so, which ones? _____
_____
_____

Did any foods provoke carb cravings, and if so, which ones? _____
_____

Were you hungry between meals and/or snacks? _____
Is your energy level high, low, or medium? _____
Do your clothes fit better? _____
Have you found yourself unable to find a low-carb meal or encoun-
tered similar challenges? If so, how did you deal with it? _____
_____
_____

Would you handle this differently in the future? If so, how? _____
_____
_____

Do you plan to change your phase and/or Net Carb level this week?
_____

Do you plan to add any new foods this week? If so, which ones?
_____
_____

Do you plan to exercise this week? If so, describe: _____
_____
_____

Do you anticipate anything interfering with eating low carb this
week? If so, how do you plan to work around it? _____
_____
_____

Describe your emotions over the last week, along with other relevant feelings and thoughts. _____
_____
_____

Date: _____

TODAY'S MEALS (including portion sizes)

Breakfast: Grams Net Carbs

_____   _____

_____   _____

_____   _____

                             Subtotal: _____

Snack:

_____   _____

Lunch:

_____   _____

_____   _____

_____   _____

_____   _____

                             Subtotal: _____

Snack:

_____   _____

Dinner:

_____   _____

_____   _____

_____   _____

_____   _____

                             Subtotal: _____

                Total grams Net Carbs: _____

Number of servings of foundation vegetables: _____

Did you take your multivitamin/mineral?   ❏ YES ❏ NO

Your omega-3 supplement?   ❏ YES ❏ NO

Your vitamin D supplement?   ❏ YES ❏ NO

Did you have the recommended salt, soy sauce,
or broth?   ❏ YES ❏ NO

Number of glasses of water: _____

TODAY'S JOURNAL

How are you doing on the diet? _____

_____

How do you feel? _____

_____

What's working for you? _____

_____

Are you experiencing any challenges and how do you plan to over-
come them? _____

_____

How do you feel about the changes you're making? _____

_____

Did you exercise today? _____
If so, what did you do and for how long? _____

_____

_____

BYE-BYE BINGES

Learn from your missteps by being scrupulously honest in
this journal. If you experience a binge-eating session, note
not just the type and amount of food you ate but also the
time of day, your hunger level before you began, and any
thoughts or emotions that may have preceded the binge. Did
you skip a meal and become ravenous? Did you consciously
place yourself in the way of temptation? Understanding why
you behaved as you did that time will help you avoid similar
situations in the future. To learn how to avoid binges, see
"Ten Unbreakable Rules" on page 33. Also, see "Short-Circuit
Binges" on page 245.

Date: _____

TODAY'S MEALS (including portion sizes)

Breakfast: Grams Net Carbs

_____   _____

_____   _____

_____   _____

                                     Subtotal: _____

Snack:

_____   _____

Lunch:

_____   _____

_____   _____

_____   _____

_____   _____

                                     Subtotal: _____

Snack:

_____   _____

Dinner:

_____   _____

_____   _____

_____   _____

_____   _____

                                     Subtotal: _____

                       Total grams Net Carbs: _____

Number of servings of foundation vegetables: _____

Did you take your multivitamin/mineral?   ❏ YES ❏ NO

Your omega-3 supplement?   ❏ YES ❏ NO

Your vitamin D supplement?   ❏ YES ❏ NO

Did you have the recommended salt, soy sauce,
or broth?   ❏ YES ❏ NO

Number of glasses of water: _____

TODAY'S JOURNAL

How are you doing on the diet? _____

_____

How do you feel? _____

_____

What's working for you? _____

_____

Are you experiencing any challenges and how do you plan to over-come them? _____

_____

How do you feel about the changes you're making? _____

_____

Did you exercise today? _____
If so, what did you do and for how long? _____

_____

_____

_____

"Motivation is what gets you started. Habit is what keeps you going."

—*Jim Ryun, athlete and politician*

Date: _____

TODAY'S MEALS (including portion sizes)

Breakfast: Grams Net Carbs

_____   _____

_____   _____

_____   _____

                          Subtotal: _____

Snack:

_____   _____

Lunch:

_____   _____

_____   _____

_____   _____

_____   _____

                          Subtotal: _____

Snack:

_____   _____

Dinner:

_____   _____

_____   _____

_____   _____

_____   _____

                          Subtotal: _____

            Total grams Net Carbs: _____

Number of servings of foundation vegetables: _____

Did you take your multivitamin/mineral?   ❏ YES ❏ NO

Your omega-3 supplement?   ❏ YES ❏ NO

Your vitamin D supplement?   ❏ YES ❏ NO

Did you have the recommended salt, soy sauce,
or broth?   ❏ YES ❏ NO

Number of glasses of water: _____

TODAY'S JOURNAL

How are you doing on the diet? _____

How do you feel? _____

What's working for you? _____

Are you experiencing any challenges and how do you plan to over-come them? _____

How do you feel about the changes you're making? _____

Did you exercise today? _____
If so, what did you do and for how long? _____
_____
_____

FOR A NEW YOU

ARE YOU DONE YET?

It takes about twenty minutes for your stomach to signal your brain that it's full. So instead of eating until you feel stuffed, stop when you feel almost full and wait twenty minutes to see if you're satisfied without eating any more. Once you distinguish habit from hunger, you may find yourself eating a bit less than you've been accustomed to without feeling empty.

Date: _____

TODAY'S MEALS (including portion sizes)

Breakfast: Grams Net Carbs

_____   _____

_____   _____

_____   _____

                                   Subtotal: _____

Snack:

_____   _____

Lunch:

_____   _____

_____   _____

_____   _____

_____   _____

                                   Subtotal: _____

Snack:

_____   _____

Dinner:

_____   _____

_____   _____

_____   _____

_____   _____

                                   Subtotal: _____

                   Total grams Net Carbs: _____

Number of servings of foundation vegetables: _____

Did you take your multivitamin/mineral?   ❑ YES   ❑ NO

Your omega-3 supplement?   ❑ YES   ❑ NO

Your vitamin D supplement?   ❑ YES   ❑ NO

Did you have the recommended salt, soy sauce,
or broth?   ❑ YES   ❑ NO

Number of glasses of water: _____

TODAY'S JOURNAL

How are you doing on the diet? _____

_____

How do you feel? _____

_____

What's working for you? _____

_____

Are you experiencing any challenges and how do you plan to over-
come them? _____

_____

How do you feel about the changes you're making? _____

_____

Did you exercise today? _____
If so, what did you do and for how long? _____

_____

_____

RECENT RESEARCH

JOURNALING YIELDS BETTER RESULTS

In a study published in the September 2012 issue of the
Journal of the Academy of Nutrition and Dietetics, researchers randomly divided 123 overweight or obese and sedentary
postmenopausal women into two groups and tracked them
for a year. Those who regularly recorded their intake in a food
diary lost about 6 more pounds than did women who didn't
keep a diary. But women who skipped meals lost about 8
fewer pounds than women who ate at least three meals a day.
One marker was consistent across both groups: daily weigh-
ins did not result in greater weight loss than weekly ones.
There is no reason men wouldn't also improve their results by
recording their food intake.

Date: _____

TODAY'S MEALS (including portion sizes)

Breakfast: Grams Net Carbs

_____   _____

_____   _____

_____   _____

                                  Subtotal: _____

Snack:

_____   _____

Lunch:

_____   _____

_____   _____

_____   _____

_____   _____

                                  Subtotal: _____

Snack:

_____   _____

Dinner:

_____   _____

_____   _____

_____   _____

_____   _____

                                  Subtotal: _____

                      Total grams Net Carbs: _____

Number of servings of foundation vegetables: _____

Did you take your multivitamin/mineral?   ❑ YES   ❑ NO

Your omega-3 supplement?   ❑ YES   ❑ NO

Your vitamin D supplement?   ❑ YES   ❑ NO

Did you have the recommended salt, soy sauce,
or broth?   ❑ YES   ❑ NO

Number of glasses of water: _____

TODAY'S JOURNAL:

How are you doing on the diet? _____

_____

How do you feel? _____

_____

What's working for you? _____

_____

Are you experiencing any challenges and how do you plan to over-
come them? _____

_____

How do you feel about the changes you're making? _____

_____

Did you exercise today? _____
If so, what did you do and for how long? _____

_____

_____

ARE MEDS HINDERING WEIGHT LOSS?

Certain drugs, including steroids, some antidepressants, insulin, and beta-blockers, can interfere with shedding pounds.
If you're taking any of these pharmaceuticals and following
Atkins to the letter but experiencing slow or little weight
loss, talk to your physician about whether you can reduce
your dosage or switch to another medication. Under no cir-
cumstances stop or reduce the level of any drug without your
doctor's approval.

Date: _____

TODAY'S MEALS (including portion sizes)

Breakfast: Grams Net Carbs

_____   _____

_____   _____

_____   _____

                              Subtotal: _____

Snack:

_____   _____

Lunch:

_____   _____

_____   _____

_____   _____

_____   _____

                              Subtotal: _____

Snack:

_____   _____

Dinner:

_____   _____

_____   _____

_____   _____

_____   _____

                              Subtotal: _____

                    Total grams Net Carbs: _____

Number of servings of foundation vegetables: _____

Did you take your multivitamin/mineral?   ❑ YES   ❑ NO

Your omega-3 supplement?   ❑ YES   ❑ NO

Your vitamin D supplement?   ❑ YES   ❑ NO

Did you have the recommended salt, soy sauce,
or broth?   ❑ YES   ❑ NO

Number of glasses of water: _____

TODAY'S JOURNAL

How are you doing on the diet? _____

_____

_____

How do you feel? _____

_____

_____

What's working for you? _____

_____

_____

Are you experiencing any challenges and how do you plan to over-
come them? _____

_____

_____

How do you feel about the changes you're making? _____

_____

_____

Did you exercise today? _____
If so, what did you do and for how long? _____

_____

_____

_____

"It's so hard when I have to, And so easy when I want to."
—*Sondra Anice Barnes, author of* Life Is the Way It Is

Date: _____

TODAY'S MEALS (including portion sizes)

Breakfast: Grams Net Carbs

_____ _____

_____ _____

_____ _____

            Subtotal: _____

Snack:

_____ _____

Lunch:

_____ _____

_____ _____

_____ _____

_____ _____

            Subtotal: _____

Snack:

_____ _____

Dinner:

_____ _____

_____ _____

_____ _____

_____ _____

            Subtotal: _____

    Total grams Net Carbs: _____

Number of servings of foundation vegetables: _____

Did you take your multivitamin/mineral?   ❏ YES   ❏ NO

Your omega-3 supplement?   ❏ YES   ❏ NO

Your vitamin D supplement?   ❏ YES   ❏ NO

Did you have the recommended salt, soy sauce,
or broth?   ❏ YES   ❏ NO

Number of glasses of water: _____

TODAY'S JOURNAL

How are you doing on the diet? _____

_____

How do you feel? _____

_____

What's working for you? _____

_____

Are you experiencing any challenges and how do you plan to over-
come them? _____

_____

How do you feel about the changes you're making? _____

_____

Did you exercise today? _____
If so, what did you do and for how long? _____

_____

_____

FOR A NEW YOU

STAR IN YOUR OWN VIDEO

A cool new app for your smartphone can be a highly moti-
vational tool as you slim down and shape up. Simply take a
photo of yourself every day or few days. (Stand in front of a
full-length mirror in the same place each time.) The Watch
Me Change Weight Loss app (www.watchmechangeapp.com/
weight-app.html) turns the sequence into a video so you can
actually see the effect of pounds disappearing over time.

WEEK 3

Two weeks under your (smaller) belt and you're probably feeling like an Atkins pro. Way to go! If you started in Induction and decided to move to Phase 2 this week, up your daily intake of Net Carbs to 25 grams. Nuts and seeds (one kind at a time) and their butters are the first thing most people add back. Your morning snack might be 24 almonds (2.7 g NC) and your afternoon snack a celery stick with a tablespoon of almond butter (1.4 g NC). If you're staying in Induction, you can also add back nuts and seeds, but keep your Net Carb count at 20 grams. In the coming weeks, you'll get to reintroduce other yummy Phase 2 foods: strawberries, raspberries, blueberries, and all their cousins, as well as cantaloupe and other melons, plus Greek yogurt and fresh cheeses.

Phase: _____ Daily Net Carb Target:_____ grams

MY CURRENT STATS
Chest: _____ inches   Waist: _____ inches
Hips: _____ inches   Upper arms: _____ inches
Thighs: _____ inches   Calves: _____ inches
Weight: _____ pounds
BMI: _____   WHR: _____

How do you feel about your results over the previous week? _____
_____
_____

Did you miss any particular foods? If so, which ones? _____
_____
_____

Did any foods provoke carb cravings, and if so, which ones? _____
_____
_____

Were you hungry between meals and/or snacks? _____
Is your energy level high, low, or medium? _____
Do your clothes fit better? _____
Have you found yourself unable to find a low-carb meal or encoun-
tered similar challenges? If so, how did you deal with it? _____
_____
_____

Would you handle this differently in the future? If so, how? _____
_____
_____

Do you plan to change phase and/or Net Carb level this week?
_____

Do you plan to add any new foods this week? If so, which ones?
_____
_____

Do you plan to exercise this week? If so, describe: _____
_____
_____

Do you anticipate anything interfering with eating low carb this
week? If so, how do you plan to work around it? _____
_____
_____

Describe your emotions over the last week, along with other relevant feelings and thoughts. _____
_____
_____
_____
_____
_____

Date: _____

TODAY'S MEALS (including portion sizes)

Breakfast: Grams Net Carbs

_____   _____

_____   _____

_____   _____

                          Subtotal: _____

Snack:

_____   _____

Lunch:

_____   _____

_____   _____

_____   _____

_____   _____

                          Subtotal: _____

Snack:

_____   _____

Dinner:

_____   _____

_____   _____

_____   _____

_____   _____

                          Subtotal: _____

            Total grams Net Carbs: _____

Number of servings of foundation vegetables: _____

Did you take your multivitamin/mineral?   ❏ YES   ❏ NO

Your omega-3 supplement?   ❏ YES   ❏ NO

Your vitamin D supplement?   ❏ YES   ❏ NO

Did you have the recommended salt, soy sauce,
or broth?   ❏ YES   ❏ NO

Number of glasses of water: _____

TODAY'S JOURNAL

How are you doing on the diet? _____

_____

How do you feel? _____

_____

What's working for you? _____

_____

Are you experiencing any challenges and how do you plan to over-
come them? _____

_____

How do you feel about the changes you're making? _____

_____

Did you exercise today? _____
If so, what did you do and for how long? _____

_____

_____

RECENT RESEARCH

A NEW WAY TO EVALUATE OBESITY

In addition to body mass index (BMI) and waist-to-hip ratio
(WHR), researchers at the City College of New York have recently introduced another indicator of obesity, which may well
become the norm. The new tool, a body shape index (ABSI),
combines your BMI and waist size. The researchers measured
the ABSI of more than 14,100 participants in the National
Health and Nutrition Examination Survey (NHANES) between 1999 and 2004. A high ABSI, which indicates excessive
belly fat, significantly increases the risk of early death. If this
new metric becomes the standard for identifying an unhealthy
body type, it would address the BMI's flaw: its inability to take
into consideration body composition. For an ABSI calculator,
go to absi-calc.appspot.com.

Date: _____

TODAY'S MEALS (including portion sizes)

Breakfast: Grams Net Carbs

_____   _____
_____   _____
_____   _____

                              Subtotal: _____

Snack:

_____   _____

Lunch:

_____   _____
_____   _____
_____   _____
_____   _____

                              Subtotal: _____

Snack:

_____   _____

Dinner:

_____   _____
_____   _____
_____   _____
_____   _____

                              Subtotal: _____
               Total grams Net Carbs: _____

Number of servings of foundation vegetables: _____

Did you take your multivitamin/mineral?   ❏ YES   ❏ NO

Your omega-3 supplement?   ❏ YES   ❏ NO

Your vitamin D supplement?   ❏ YES   ❏ NO

Did you have the recommended salt, soy sauce,
or broth?   ❏ YES   ❏ NO

Number of glasses of water: _____

TODAY'S JOURNAL

How are you doing on the diet? _____

_____

How do you feel? _____

_____

What's working for you? _____

_____

Are you experiencing any challenges and how do you plan to over-
come them? _____

_____

How do you feel about the changes you're making? _____

_____

Did you exercise today? _____
If so, what did you do and for how long? _____

_____

_____

FOR A NEW YOU

ACCENTUATE THE POSITIVE

Instead of beating yourself up because your body doesn't re-
semble the unrealistic body images projected in the media,
understand that your physical self is as unique as your
personality. Use this journal to record the things you like
about yourself, whether physical attributes—your blue eyes,
wavy hair, or athletic prowess—or those unrelated to your
appearance—your deep friendships, parenting skills, way
with plants, batting average, or whatever else you're proud of.
The more you see yourself as a successful human being, the
more successful you'll be in your efforts to achieve the best
version of the body you were born with.

Date: _____

TODAY'S MEALS (including portion sizes)

Breakfast: Grams Net Carbs

_____ _____

_____ _____

_____ _____

                        Subtotal: _____

Snack:

_____ _____

Lunch:

_____ _____

_____ _____

_____ _____

_____ _____

                        Subtotal: _____

Snack:

_____ _____

Dinner:

_____ _____

_____ _____

_____ _____

_____ _____

                        Subtotal: _____

            Total grams Net Carbs: _____

Number of servings of foundation vegetables: _____

Did you take your multivitamin/mineral?   ❏ YES ❏ NO

Your omega-3 supplement?   ❏ YES ❏ NO

Your vitamin D supplement?   ❏ YES ❏ NO

Did you have the recommended salt, soy sauce,
or broth?   ❏ YES ❏ NO

Number of glasses of water: _____

TODAY'S JOURNAL

How are you doing on the diet? _____

_____

_____

How do you feel? _____

_____

_____

What's working for you? _____

_____

Are you experiencing any challenges and how do you plan to over-
come them?

_____

_____

How do you feel about the changes you're making? _____

_____

_____

Did you exercise today? _____
If so, what did you do and for how long? _____

_____

_____

_____

"Motivation is the single most important factor in any sort
of success."

—*Sir Edmund Hillary, New Zealand mountaineer who first*
scaled Mount Everest along with his Nepalese Sherpa guide

Date: _____

TODAY'S MEALS (including portion sizes)

Breakfast: Grams Net Carbs

_____ _____

_____ _____

_____ _____

Subtotal: _____

Snack:

_____ _____

Lunch:

_____ _____

_____ _____

_____ _____

_____ _____

Subtotal: _____

Snack:

_____ _____

Dinner:

_____ _____

_____ _____

_____ _____

_____ _____

Subtotal: _____

Total grams Net Carbs: _____

Number of servings of foundation vegetables: _____

Did you take your multivitamin/mineral?   ❑ YES   ❑ NO

Your omega-3 supplement?   ❑ YES   ❑ NO

Your vitamin D supplement?   ❑ YES   ❑ NO

Did you have the recommended salt, soy sauce,
or broth?   ❑ YES   ❑ NO

Number of glasses of water: _____

TODAY'S JOURNAL

How are you doing on the diet? _____

_____

How do you feel? _____

_____

What's working for you? _____

_____

Are you experiencing any challenges and how do you plan to over-
come them? _____

_____

How do you feel about the changes you're making? _____

_____

Did you exercise today? _____
If so, what did you do and for how long? _____

_____

_____

FOR A NEW YOU

HUNTING DOWN HIDDEN SUGARS

Added sugar and all its empty carbs (see "What and Where
Are Added Sugars?" on page 16) pop up in many processed
foods. Not surprisingly, they're in most baked goods and des-
serts, but other prime offenders include breakfast cereals,
bottled ice teas, pasta sauces, canned soups, bottled salad
dressings, ketchup, and barbecue sauce. Always read labels
scrupulously.

Date: _____

TODAY'S MEALS (including portion sizes)

Breakfast: Grams Net Carbs

_____   _____

_____   _____

_____   _____

                                    Subtotal: _____

Snack:

_____   _____

Lunch:

_____   _____

_____   _____

_____   _____

_____   _____

                                    Subtotal: _____

Snack:

_____   _____

Dinner:

_____   _____

_____   _____

_____   _____

_____   _____

                                    Subtotal: _____

                        Total grams Net Carbs: _____

Number of servings of foundation vegetables: _____

Did you take your multivitamin/mineral?   ❏ YES ❏ NO

Your omega-3 supplement?   ❏ YES ❏ NO

Your vitamin D supplement?   ❏ YES ❏ NO

Did you have the recommended salt, soy sauce,
or broth?   ❏ YES ❏ NO

Number of glasses of water: _____

TODAY'S JOURNAL

How are you doing on the diet? _____

_____

How do you feel? _____

_____

What's working for you? _____

_____

Are you experiencing any challenges and how do you plan to over-
come them? _____

_____

How do you feel about the changes you're making? _____

_____

Did you exercise today? _____
If so, what did you do and for how long? _____

_____

_____

LOW-CARB DIET BURNS
THE MOST CALORIES

A 2012 study published in the *Journal of the American Medical Association* revealed that people who were trying to maintain their weight loss burned about 300 more calories a day eating a diet modeled on the Induction phase of Atkins than they did eating a low-fat diet. Moreover, on the low-carb diet they experienced positive results such as increased HDL ("good") cholesterol, lowered triglycerides, reduced inflammation, and improved insulin sensitivity. According to the researchers, "These findings suggest that a strategy to reduce glycemic load rather than dietary fat may be advantageous for weight-loss maintenance and cardiovascular disease prevention."

Date: _____

TODAY'S MEALS (including portion sizes)

Breakfast: Grams Net Carbs

_____   _____

_____   _____

_____   _____

                                Subtotal: _____

Snack:

_____   _____

Lunch:

_____   _____

_____   _____

_____   _____

_____   _____

                                Subtotal: _____

Snack:

_____   _____

Dinner:

_____   _____

_____   _____

_____   _____

_____   _____

                                Subtotal: _____

                    Total grams Net Carbs: _____

Number of servings of foundation vegetables: _____

Did you take your multivitamin/mineral?   ❏ YES   ❏ NO

Your omega-3 supplement?   ❏ YES   ❏ NO

Your vitamin D supplement?   ❏ YES   ❏ NO

Did you have the recommended salt, soy sauce,

or broth?   ❏ YES   ❏ NO

Number of glasses of water: _____

TODAY'S JOURNAL

How are you doing on the diet? _____

_____

How do you feel? _____

_____

What's working for you? _____

_____

Are you experiencing any challenges and how do you plan to over-
come them? _____

_____

How do you feel about the changes you're making? _____

_____

Did you exercise today? _____
If so, what did you do and for how long? _____

_____

_____

FOR A NEW YOU

GET MOVING TO GET MOTIVATED

Far from exhausting yourself, moderate physical activity—
such as jogging or taking a strength-training class at the
gym—is energizing and lifts your mood so that you'll feel
more motivated to stick with your weight loss program.
That's one more reason why exercising and watching your
food intake are a natural combo.

Date: _____

TODAY'S MEALS (including portion sizes)

Breakfast: Grams Net Carbs

_____   _____

_____   _____

_____   _____

Subtotal: _____

Snack:

_____   _____

Lunch:

_____   _____

_____   _____

_____   _____

_____   _____

Subtotal: _____

Snack:

_____   _____

Dinner:

_____   _____

_____   _____

_____   _____

_____   _____

Subtotal: _____

Total grams Net Carbs: _____

Number of servings of foundation vegetables: _____

Did you take your multivitamin/mineral?   ❏ YES ❏ NO

Your omega-3 supplement?   ❏ YES ❏ NO

Your vitamin D supplement?   ❏ YES ❏ NO

Did you have the recommended salt, soy sauce,
or broth?   ❏ YES ❏ NO

Number of glasses of water: _____

TODAY'S JOURNAL

How are you doing on the diet? _____

_____

How do you feel? _____

_____

What's working for you? _____

_____

Are you experiencing any challenges and how do you plan to over-
come them?

_____

_____

How do you feel about the changes you're making? _____

_____

_____

Did you exercise today? _____
If so, what did you do and for how long? _____

_____

_____

_____

"The secret of discipline is motivation. When a man is
sufficiently motivated, discipline will take care of itself."

—*Albert Einstein*

WEEK 4

If you've already banished a significant number of pounds and inches, bravo! If you're not pleased with the pace of weight loss, now is the time for a reality check. First of all, if you're middle aged or older, insulin resistant, or sedentary, it will take longer to slim down. If you're younger and active, you may need to make some course corrections. Are you eating more than 6 ounces of protein at a meal? Cut back. Holding back on fat? Include it in your meals. Or you may simply be eating too much. If you're just estimating Net Carbs, use a carb counter. Are you eating enough foundation vegetables? Their fiber and water content fills you up so you're likely to eat less. Are you really getting at least eight 8-ounce glasses of water a day, consuming hidden carbs in condiments, using more than three packets of noncaloric sweeteners a day, skipping meals, or going too long between a meal or snack and the next meal? Review your habits carefully and you'll probably come up with the explanation for your frustration. Adding moderately intense exercise, if you have not already done so, may also pick up the pace.

Phase: _____ Daily Net Carb Target: _____ grams

MY CURRENT STATS

Chest: _____ inches   Waist: _____ inches

Hips: _____ inches   Upper arms: _____ inches

Thighs: _____ inches   Calves: _____ inches

Weight: _____ pounds

BMI: _____   WHR: _____

How do you feel about your results over the previous week? _____

_____

Did you miss any particular foods? If so, which ones? _____

_____

Did any foods provoke carb cravings, and if so, which ones? _____

_____

Were you hungry between meals and/or snacks? _____

Is your energy level high, low, or medium? _____

Do your clothes fit better? _____

Have you ever found yourself unable to find a low-carb meal or encountered similar challenges? If so, how did you deal with it? _____

_____

Would you handle this differently in the future? If so, how? _____

_____

Do you plan to change the phase and/or Net Carb level this week?

_____

Do you plan to add any new foods this week? If so, which ones?

_____

Do you plan to exercise this week? If so, describe:_____

_____

Do you anticipate anything interfering with eating low carb this week? If so, how do you plan to work around it? _____

_____

Describe your emotions over the last week, along with other relevant feelings and thoughts. _____

_____

_____

_____

Date: _____

TODAY'S MEALS (including portion sizes)

Breakfast: Grams Net Carbs

_____   _____

_____   _____

_____   _____

                                 Subtotal: _____

Snack:

_____   _____

Lunch:

_____   _____

_____   _____

_____   _____

_____   _____

                                 Subtotal: _____

Snack:

_____   _____

Dinner:

_____   _____

_____   _____

_____   _____

_____   _____

                                 Subtotal: _____

                    Total grams Net Carbs: _____

Number of servings of foundation vegetables: _____

Did you take your multivitamin/mineral?   ❑ YES   ❑ NO

Your omega-3 supplement?   ❑ YES   ❑ NO

Your vitamin D supplement?   ❑ YES   ❑ NO

Did you have the recommended salt, soy sauce,
or broth?   ❑ YES   ❑ NO

Number of glasses of water: _____

TODAY'S JOURNAL

How are you doing on the diet? _____
_____

How do you feel? _____
_____

What's working for you? _____
_____

Are you experiencing any challenges and how do you plan to over-
come them? _____
_____

How do you feel about the changes you're making? _____
_____

Did you exercise today? _____
If so, what did you do and for how long? _____
_____
_____

FOR A NEW YOU

MIND THE CLOCK

Establishing regular eating habits will help you eat better and
resist the temptation of sugar-filled or other high-carb foods.
Try to eat your three main meals and two snacks at roughly
the same time each day. If you know you may not be able to
have a meal, be prepared with a snack that includes protein
and fat.

Date: _____

TODAY'S MEALS (including portion sizes)

Breakfast: Grams Net Carbs

_____   _____

_____   _____

_____   _____

                               Subtotal: _____

Snack:

_____   _____

Lunch:

_____   _____

_____   _____

_____   _____

_____   _____

                               Subtotal: _____

Snack:

_____   _____

Dinner:

_____   _____

_____   _____

_____   _____

_____   _____

                               Subtotal: _____

                  Total grams Net Carbs: _____

Number of servings of foundation vegetables: _____

Did you take your multivitamin/mineral?   ❏ YES ❏ NO

Your omega-3 supplement?   ❏ YES ❏ NO

Your vitamin D supplement?   ❏ YES ❏ NO

Did you have the recommended salt, soy sauce,
or broth?   ❏ YES ❏ NO

Number of glasses of water: _____

TODAY'S JOURNAL

How are you doing on the diet? _____

_____

How do you feel? _____

_____

What's working for you? _____

_____

Are you experiencing any challenges and how do you plan to over-
come them? _____

_____

How do you feel about the changes you're making? _____

_____

Did you exercise today? _____
If so, what did you do and for how long? _____

_____

_____

RECENT RESEARCH

SLEEP OFF EXCESS WEIGHT

People who get more sleep tend to have a lower BMI than
people who skimp on sleep. Now a 2012 study at the University of Washington Medicine Sleep Center, published
in the journal *Sleep*, suggests that more sleep can actually
override a genetic propensity to being overweight. By using
pairs of identical and fraternal twins, neurologist Nathanial
Watson found that identical twins, who have the same genetic
makeup, display weight differences based on the amount of
time each sleeps. With less than seven hours of sleep a night,
one twin's BMI tends to be higher than the other. This suggests that the less sleep one gets, the more genes contribute
to determining weight, but with more sleep, the influence of
genes on weight is reduced.

Date: _____

TODAY'S MEALS (including portion sizes)

Breakfast: Grams Net Carbs

_____   _____

_____   _____

_____   _____

                                     Subtotal: _____

Snack:

_____   _____

Lunch:

_____   _____

_____   _____

_____   _____

_____   _____

                                     Subtotal: _____

Snack:

_____   _____

Dinner:

_____   _____

_____   _____

_____   _____

_____   _____

                                     Subtotal: _____

                          Total grams Net Carbs: _____

Number of servings of foundation vegetables: _____

Did you take your multivitamin/mineral?   ❏ YES   ❏ NO

Your omega-3 supplement?   ❏ YES   ❏ NO

Your vitamin D supplement?   ❏ YES   ❏ NO

Did you have the recommended salt, soy sauce,
or broth?   ❏ YES   ❏ NO

Number of glasses of water: _____

TODAY'S JOURNAL

How are you doing on the diet? _____

_____

How do you feel? _____

_____

What's working for you? _____

_____

Are you experiencing any challenges and how do you plan to over-
come them? _____

_____

How do you feel about the changes you're making? _____

_____

Did you exercise today? _____
If so, what did you do and for how long? _____

_____

_____

FOR A NEW YOU

TAKE AN EXERCISE BREAK

Exercising regularly is key to getting results, but don't let your
newfound enthusiasm increase the risk of hurting yourself or
overdoing it. Any fitness trainer will tell you that it's important to take at least one or two days off a week to allow your
body to rest and recover between exercise bouts. By not over-
exercising, you're far more likely to get into a regular pattern
without injuring yourself or becoming discouraged.

Date: _____

TODAY'S MEALS (including portion sizes)

Breakfast: Grams Net Carbs

_____   _____
_____   _____
_____   _____

                              Subtotal: _____

Snack:

_____   _____

Lunch:

_____   _____
_____   _____
_____   _____
_____   _____

                              Subtotal: _____

Snack:

_____   _____

Dinner:

_____   _____
_____   _____
_____   _____
_____   _____

                              Subtotal: _____
               Total grams Net Carbs: _____

Number of servings of foundation vegetables: _____

Did you take your multivitamin/mineral?   ❏ YES   ❏ NO

Your omega-3 supplement?   ❏ YES   ❏ NO

Your vitamin D supplement?   ❏ YES   ❏ NO

Did you have the recommended salt, soy sauce,
or broth?   ❏ YES   ❏ NO

Number of glasses of water: _____

TODAY'S JOURNAL

How are you doing on the diet? _____
_____
_____

How do you feel? _____
_____
_____

What's working for you? _____
_____
_____

Are you experiencing any challenges and how do you plan to over-
come them? _____
_____
_____

How do you feel about the changes you're making? _____
_____
_____

Did you exercise today? _____
If so, what did you do and for how long? _____
_____
_____
_____

"The vision must be followed by the venture. It is not enough to
stare up the steps, we must step up the stairs."

—*Vance Havner, Baptist minister and inspirational author*

WEEK 1	WEEK 2	WEEK 3	**WEEK 4**

DAY 1	DAY 2	DAY 3	DAY 4	**DAY 5**	DAY 6	DAY 7

Date: _____

TODAY'S MEALS (including portion sizes)

Breakfast: Grams Net Carbs

_____   _____

_____   _____

_____   _____

Subtotal: _____

Snack:

_____   _____

Lunch:

_____   _____

_____   _____

_____   _____

_____   _____

Subtotal: _____

Snack:

_____   _____

Dinner:

_____   _____

_____   _____

_____   _____

_____   _____

Subtotal: _____

Total grams Net Carbs: _____

Number of servings of foundation vegetables: _____

Did you take your multivitamin/mineral?   ❏ YES ❏ NO

Your omega-3 supplement?   ❏ YES ❏ NO

Your vitamin D supplement?   ❏ YES ❏ NO

Did you have the recommended salt, soy sauce,
or broth?   ❏ YES ❏ NO

Number of glasses of water: _____

TODAY'S JOURNAL

How are you doing on the diet? _____

_____

How do you feel? _____

_____

What's working for you? _____

_____

Are you experiencing any challenges and how do you plan to over-
come them? _____

_____

How do you feel about the changes you're making? _____

_____

Did you exercise today? _____
If so, what did you do and for how long? _____

_____

_____

FOR A NEW YOU

THE NOSE KNOWS

The scent of bread baking or the sweet perfume of sticky
buns don't just test resolve; the sight or scent of food can also
stimulate your appetite and cause cravings. While you can't
control your body's automatic response, you can stay away
from situations that expose you to foods that trigger such a
reaction. The next time a friend asks to meet you at a coffee
shop known for its delectable baked goods or a pizzeria, come
up with another, safer suggestion.

Date: _____

TODAY'S MEALS (including portion sizes)

Breakfast: Grams Net Carbs

_____   _____

_____   _____

_____   _____

                        Subtotal: _____

Snack:

_____

Lunch:

_____   _____

_____   _____

_____   _____

_____   _____

                        Subtotal: _____

Snack:

_____

Dinner:

_____   _____

_____   _____

_____   _____

_____   _____

                        Subtotal: _____

            Total grams Net Carbs: _____

Number of servings of foundation vegetables: _____

Did you take your multivitamin/mineral?   ❑ YES   ❑ NO

Your omega-3 supplement?   ❑ YES   ❑ NO

Your vitamin D supplement?   ❑ YES   ❑ NO

Did you have the recommended salt, soy sauce,
or broth?   ❑ YES   ❑ NO

Number of glasses of water: _____

TODAY'S JOURNAL

How are you doing on the diet? _____
_____

How do you feel? _____
_____

What's working for you? _____
_____

Are you experiencing any challenges and how do you plan to over-
come them? _____
_____

How do you feel about the changes you're making? _____
_____

Did you exercise today? _____
If so, what did you do and for how long? _____
_____
_____

RECENT RESEARCH

PEPPER MAY AID WEIGHT LOSS

It can't hurt to give your meals an extra grind of black pepper. Piperine, the component in black pepper that sharpens
the taste of savory foods, may be a new tool in the battle
against obesity and related diseases. According to researchers at Seoul's Sejong University in a 2012 study published in
the *Journal of Agricultural and Food Chemistry*, piperine plays
interference in the body, blocking the generation of new fat
cells. The researchers had previously found that piperine can
reduce the levels of fat in the bloodstream. Traditional East-
ern medicine has long used black pepper to treat an array of
health disorders, including pain and inflammation.

Date: _____

TODAY'S MEALS (including portion sizes)

Breakfast: Grams Net Carbs

_____   _____

_____   _____

_____   _____

                                   Subtotal: _____

Snack:

_____   _____

Lunch:

_____   _____

_____   _____

_____   _____

_____   _____

                                   Subtotal: _____

Snack:

_____   _____

Dinner:

_____   _____

_____   _____

_____   _____

_____   _____

                                   Subtotal: _____

                        Total grams Net Carbs: _____

Number of servings of foundation vegetables: _____

Did you take your multivitamin/mineral?   ❏ YES ❏ NO

Your omega-3 supplement?   ❏ YES ❏ NO

Your vitamin D supplement?   ❏ YES ❏ NO

Did you have the recommended salt, soy sauce,
or broth?   ❏ YES ❏ NO

Number of glasses of water: _____

TODAY'S JOURNAL

How are you doing on the diet? _____

_____

How do you feel? _____

_____

What's working for you? _____

_____

Are you experiencing any challenges and how do you plan to over-
come them? _____

_____

How do you feel about the changes you're making? _____

_____

Did you exercise today? _____
If so, what did you do and for how long? _____

_____

_____

FOR A NEW YOU

THINK CONSTRUCTIVELY

Jot down in this journal the bad thoughts that sneak into your
mind when you're feeling sorry for yourself. Then turn that
sentence around. If you wrote, "I'm so heavy, I will never have
a boyfriend (or girlfriend)," instead write, "I know I'm lovable
because my parents, my sister, and my nephew all love me,
and I will find a partner who also loves me." Or instead of "I
know this diet will fail, just as the others have before," write,
"This time I'm going to be successful because now I can see
that I went back to my old bad habits after losing weight, and
now I understand I must make a lifestyle change."

WEEK 5

If you're already walking regularly or otherwise being physically active, you're on the right track, pun intended. But if you felt that starting an exercise program at the same time you began a new way of eating was too much too soon, that's perfectly understandable. Now that you're in the Atkins groove, it would be a super time to add fitness to your routine. Exercise may or may not enhance your weight loss, but it will definitely help firm your body and make you feel good about yourself. You can do these moves while watching television: right and left leg lifts as you sit on the sofa, pushups supporting yourself on the back of a sofa or chair—they're much easier to do than on floor pushups—and "bicycle" while sitting on the edge of the seat and leaning back without touching the back. During the ads, do standing lunges (right and left leg) and end with some squats. If these moves are unfamiliar, check them out on YouTube and other online sites. At this point, most people don't need to continue to increase their sodium intake with broth, salt, or soy sauce to avoid certain symptoms, but continue to do so if you wish.

Phase: _____ Daily Net Carb Target: _____ grams

MY CURRENT STATS

Chest: _____ inches   Waist: _____ inches
Hips: _____ inches   Upper arms: _____ inches
Thighs: _____ inches   Calves: _____ inches
Weight: _____ pounds
BMI: _____   WHR: _____

How do you feel about your results over the previous week? _____
_____

Did you miss any particular foods? If so, which ones? _____
_____

Did any foods provoke carb cravings, and if so, which ones? _____
_____

Were you hungry between meals and/or snacks? _____
Is your energy level high, low, or medium? _____
Do your clothes fit better? _____
Have you found yourself unable to find a low-carb meal or encoun-
tered similar challenges? If so, how did you deal with it? _____
_____

Would you handle this differently in the future? If so, how? _____
_____

Do you plan to change the phase and/or Net Carb level this week?
_____

Do you plan to add any new foods this week? If so, which ones?
_____

Do you plan to exercise this week? If so, describe: _____
_____

Do you anticipate anything interfering with eating low carb this
week? If so, how do you plan to work around it? _____
_____

Describe your emotions over the last week, along with other relevant feelings and thoughts. _____
_____
_____
_____

Date: _____

TODAY'S MEALS (including portion sizes)

Breakfast: Grams Net Carbs

_____   _____

_____   _____

_____   _____

                                    Subtotal: _____

Snack:

_____   _____

Lunch:

_____   _____

_____   _____

_____   _____

_____   _____

                                    Subtotal: _____

Snack:

_____   _____

Dinner:

_____   _____

_____   _____

_____   _____

_____   _____

                                    Subtotal: _____

                     Total grams Net Carbs: _____

Number of servings of foundation vegetables: _____

Did you take your multivitamin/mineral?   ❏ YES ❏ NO

Your omega-3 supplement?   ❏ YES ❏ NO

Your vitamin D supplement?   ❏ YES ❏ NO

Number of glasses of water: _____

TODAY'S JOURNAL

How are you doing on the diet? _____
_____
_____

How do you feel? _____
_____
_____

What's working for you? _____
_____

Are you experiencing any challenges and how do you plan to overcome them? _____
_____
_____

How do you feel about the changes you're making? _____
_____
_____

Did you exercise today? _____
If so, what did you do and for how long? _____
_____
_____
_____

"Start by doing what's necessary; then do what's possible; and suddenly you are doing the impossible."

—*Saint Francis of Assisi*

Date: _____

TODAY'S MEALS (including portion sizes)

Breakfast: Grams Net Carbs

_____   _____

_____   _____

_____   _____

                                    Subtotal: _____

Snack:

_____   _____

Lunch:

_____   _____

_____   _____

_____   _____

_____   _____

                                    Subtotal: _____

Snack:

_____   _____

Dinner:

_____   _____

_____   _____

_____   _____

_____   _____

                                    Subtotal: _____

                        Total grams Net Carbs: _____

Number of servings of foundation vegetables: _____

Did you take your multivitamin/mineral?   ❑ YES   ❑ NO

Your omega-3 supplement?   ❑ YES   ❑ NO

Your vitamin D supplement?   ❑ YES   ❑ NO

Number of glasses of water: _____

TODAY'S JOURNAL

How are you doing on the diet? _____

_____

How do you feel? _____

_____

What's working for you? _____

_____

Are you experiencing any challenges and how do you plan to over-
come them? _____

_____

How do you feel about the changes you're making? _____

_____

Did you exercise today? _____
If so, what did you do and for how long? _____

_____

_____

THE ATKINS PANTRY

It's easy to do Atkins when you have the right food on hand,
particularly fresh vegetables and chicken, fish, burgers, and
eggs, plus staples such as olive oil. It's also smart to have some
nonperishables available in the pantry so when the fridge is
bare you don't have to make an emergency run to the store.
With chicken, tuna, or salmon in cans or vacuum bags, a can
of tomatoes, and some marinated artichoke hearts and marinated roasted red peppers on hand, you can throw together
a tasty Atkins-friendly meal in a few minutes. For a more
extensive list of pantry items to have at the ready, check out
The New Atkins Kitchen in *The New Atkins for a New You
Cookbook*.

Date: _____

TODAY'S MEALS (including portion sizes)

Breakfast: Grams Net Carbs

_____   _____

_____   _____

_____   _____

                            Subtotal: _____

Snack:

_____   _____

Lunch:

_____   _____

_____   _____

_____   _____

_____   _____

                            Subtotal: _____

Snack:

Dinner:

_____   _____

_____   _____

_____   _____

_____   _____

                            Subtotal: _____

              Total grams Net Carbs: _____

Number of servings of foundation vegetables: _____

Did you take your multivitamin/mineral?   ❏ YES   ❏ NO

Your omega-3 supplement?   ❏ YES   ❏ NO

Your vitamin D supplement?   ❏ YES   ❏ NO

Number of glasses of water: _____

TODAY'S JOURNAL

How are you doing on the diet? _____

_____

How do you feel? _____

_____

What's working for you? _____

_____

Are you experiencing any challenges and how do you plan to overcome them? _____

_____

How do you feel about the changes you're making? _____

_____

Did you exercise today? _____
If so, what did you do and for how long? _____

_____

_____

RECENT RESEARCH

LOW CARB RESULTS IN LESS HUNGER THAN LOW FAT

A 2011 study by researchers at Temple University and other institutions published in *Obesity* compared the effects of following either a low-carb or a low-fat diet on food cravings, food preferences, and appetite over two and a half years. Individuals in the low-carb group reported that they were less likely to crave starchy and sugary foods than did individuals on the low-fat diet. Meanwhile, the low-fat dieters found that their cravings for high-fat foods were more diminished than those of the low-carb dieters. Overall, low-carbers were less bothered by hunger than low-fat dieters, and men in both groups reported greater decreases in appetite than women.

Date: _____

TODAY'S MEALS (including portion sizes)

Breakfast: Grams Net Carbs

_____   _____

_____   _____

_____   _____

                                  Subtotal: _____

Snack:

_____

Lunch:

_____   _____

_____   _____

_____   _____

_____   _____

                                  Subtotal: _____

Snack:

_____

Dinner:

_____   _____

_____   _____

_____   _____

_____   _____

                                  Subtotal: _____

                    Total grams Net Carbs: _____

Number of servings of foundation vegetables: _____

Did you take your multivitamin/mineral?   ❏ YES   ❏ NO

Your omega-3 supplement?   ❏ YES   ❏ NO

Your vitamin D supplement?   ❏ YES   ❏ NO

Number of glasses of water: _____

TODAY'S JOURNAL

How are you doing on the diet? _____

_____

How do you feel? _____

_____

What's working for you? _____

_____

Are you experiencing any challenges and how do you plan to over-come them? _____

_____

How do you feel about the changes you're making? _____

_____

Did you exercise today? _____
If so, what did you do and for how long? _____

_____

_____

FOR A NEW YOU

FOR A NEW YOU

Before making lunch or dinner plans—whether you're talking a burger joint or a fine restaurant—go online, where chains and many other establishments now display their menus. You may decide that the restaurant is a minefield of high-carb meals and decide on another place. But don't stop there. Once you choose the venue, decide which menu items you'll be ordering and stick with them.

Date: _____

TODAY'S MEALS (including portion sizes)

Breakfast: Grams Net Carbs
_____   _____
_____   _____
_____   _____
                          Subtotal: _____

Snack:
_____   _____

Lunch:
_____   _____
_____   _____
_____   _____
_____   _____
                          Subtotal: _____

Snack:
_____   _____

Dinner:
_____   _____
_____   _____
_____   _____
_____   _____
                          Subtotal: _____
           Total grams Net Carbs: _____

Number of servings of foundation vegetables: _____
Did you take your multivitamin/mineral?   ❏ YES   ❏ NO
Your omega-3 supplement?   ❏ YES   ❏ NO
Your vitamin D supplement?   ❏ YES   ❏ NO
Number of glasses of water: _____

TODAY'S JOURNAL

How are you doing on the diet? _____

_____

_____

How do you feel? _____

_____

_____

What's working for you? _____

_____

_____

Are you experiencing any challenges and how do you plan to over-come them? _____

_____

_____

_____

How do you feel about the changes you're making? _____

_____

_____

Did you exercise today? _____
If so, what did you do and for how long? _____

_____

_____

_____

> "When there is a start to be made, don't step over! Start where you are."
>
> —*Edgar Cayce, psychic and theologian*

Date: _____

TODAY'S MEALS (including portion sizes)

Breakfast: Grams Net Carbs

_____   _____

_____   _____

_____   _____

Subtotal: _____

Snack:

_____   _____

Lunch:

_____   _____

_____   _____

_____   _____

_____   _____

Subtotal: _____

Snack:

_____   _____

Dinner:

_____   _____

_____   _____

_____   _____

_____   _____

Subtotal: _____

Total grams Net Carbs: _____

Number of servings of foundation vegetables: _____

Did you take your multivitamin/mineral?   ❑ YES   ❑ NO

Your omega-3 supplement?   ❑ YES   ❑ NO

Your vitamin D supplement?   ❑ YES   ❑ NO

Number of glasses of water: _____

TODAY'S JOURNAL

How are you doing on the diet? _____
_____

How do you feel? _____
_____

What's working for you? _____
_____

Are you experiencing any challenges and how do you plan to over-
come them? _____
_____

How do you feel about the changes you're making? _____
_____

Did you exercise today? _____
If so, what did you do and for how long? _____
_____
_____

MAKE EXERCISE A SOCIAL OCCASION

Knowing that someone is waiting for you at the corner or by
the elevator is a powerful motivator to stick with your fitness goals. Once you get in the habit of exercise, you'll find it
easier to motivate yourself, but until that happens, meeting a
friend for a walk or a jog several times a week at a designated
time and place can be a big help. Or join a health club with
a workmate—you may be able to get a discount—and com-
mit to going several times at lunchtime or after work to get
your money's worth. How about signing up with a buddy or
your partner for classes—doubles tennis, Zumba, Pilates, or
whatever—and then go a couple of times a week?

Date: _____

TODAY'S MEALS (including portion sizes)

Breakfast: Grams Net Carbs

_____   _____

_____   _____

_____   _____

Subtotal: _____

Snack:

_____   _____

Lunch:

_____   _____

_____   _____

_____   _____

_____   _____

Subtotal: _____

Snack:

_____   _____

Dinner:

_____   _____

_____   _____

_____   _____

_____   _____

Subtotal: _____

Total grams Net Carbs: _____

Number of servings of foundation vegetables: _____

Did you take your multivitamin/mineral?   ❏ YES   ❏ NO

Your omega-3 supplement?   ❏ YES   ❏ NO

Your vitamin D supplement?   ❏ YES   ❏ NO

Number of glasses of water: _____

TODAY'S JOURNAL

How are you doing on the diet? _____

_____

How do you feel? _____

_____

What's working for you? _____

_____

Are you experiencing any challenges and how do you plan to overcome them? _____

_____

How do you feel about the changes you're making? _____

_____

Did you exercise today? _____
If so, what did you do and for how long? _____

_____

_____

RECENT RESEARCH

MULTIPLE STUDIES SHOW ATKINS SAFE AND EFFECTIVE

A 2012 meta-analysis study done at Duke University Medical Center and published in *Obesity Reviews* looked at twenty-three published articles on seventeen different clinical studies comparing the Atkins Diet to other diets. Atkins was shown to be safe and effective for both weight loss and cardiovascular health. Specifically, the low-carb approach was associated with significant decreases in body weight, BMI, waist size, blood pressure, triglycerides, fasting blood sugar, glycated hemoglobin, insulin, and C-reactive protein (a marker of inflammation), as well as an increase in HDL ("good") cholesterol. LDL cholesterol did not change significantly.

WEEK 6

Give yourself a pat on the back for your good work on the program. After five weeks you're well on the way to developing new and healthy habits. If you started Atkins in Phase 1, Induction, and are still hanging out there, give some thought as to whether you should continue to stay here any longer. It's perfectly fine to do so if you have a lot of weight to lose. But if you're within 15 pounds of your goal weight or are getting bored with the food choices in Phase 1— which could lead to temptation and noncompliance—it's time to move on to Phase 2, Ongoing Weight Loss (OWL), where most people peel off the majority of their excess pounds. Remember, the real point of the four-phase program is to gradually acclimate yourself to a new, permanent way of eating—and staying too long in Induction can become a crutch. Likewise, if you're already in OWL but homing in on the last 10 pounds of your goal weight, it would be a good idea to move directly to Phase 3, Pre-Maintenance.

Phase: _____ Daily Net Carb Target:_____ grams

MY CURRENT STATS

Chest: _____ inches Waist: _____ inches

Hips: _____ inches Upper arms: _____ inches

Thighs: _____ inches Calves: _____ inches

Weight: _____ pounds

BMI: _____ WHR: _____

How do you feel about your results over the previous week? _____
_____
_____

Did you miss any particular foods? If so, which ones? _____
_____
_____

Did any foods provoke carb cravings, and if so, which ones? _____
_____
_____

Were you hungry between meals and/or snacks? _____
Is your energy level high, low, or medium? _____
Do your clothes fit better? _____
Have you found yourself unable to find a low-carb meal or encoun-
tered similar challenges? If so, how did you deal with it? _____
_____
_____

Would you handle this differently in the future? If so, how? _____
_____
_____

Do you plan to change the phase and/or Net Carb level this week?
_____

Do you plan to add any new foods this week? If so, which ones? ___
_____
_____

Do you plan to exercise this week? If so, describe: _____
_____
_____

Do you anticipate anything interfering with eating low carb this
week? If so, how do you plan to work around it? _____
_____
_____

Describe your emotions over the last week, along with other relevant feelings and thoughts. _____
_____
_____

Date: _____

TODAY'S MEALS (including portion sizes)

Breakfast: Grams Net Carbs

_____   _____
_____   _____
_____   _____
                                 Subtotal: _____

Snack:

_____   _____

Lunch:

_____   _____
_____   _____
_____   _____
_____   _____
                                 Subtotal: _____

Snack:

_____   _____

Dinner:

_____   _____
_____   _____
_____   _____
_____   _____
                                 Subtotal: _____
                    Total grams Net Carbs: _____

Number of servings of foundation vegetables: _____

Did you take your multivitamin/mineral?   ❑ YES ❑ NO

Your omega-3 supplement?   ❑ YES ❑ NO

Your vitamin D supplement?   ❑ YES ❑ NO

Number of glasses of water: _____

TODAY'S JOURNAL

How are you doing on the diet? _____

_____

How do you feel? _____

_____

What's working for you? _____

_____

Are you experiencing any challenges and how do you plan to overcome them? _____

_____

How do you feel about the changes you're making? _____

_____

Did you exercise today? _____
If so, what did you do and for how long? _____

_____

_____

FOR A NEW YOU

KEEP SIPPING

To avoid coming up short fluid-wise at the end of the day, keep a 32-ounce bottle of water by your side and sip it throughout the morning. After lunch, refill the bottle and consume the contents by dinnertime. That way, you'll be well hydrated without having to visit the bathroom during the night.

Date: _____

TODAY'S MEALS (including portion sizes)

Breakfast: Grams Net Carbs

_____   _____

_____   _____

_____   _____

                        Subtotal: _____

Snack:

_____   _____

Lunch:

_____   _____

_____   _____

_____   _____

                        Subtotal: _____

Snack:

_____   _____

Dinner:

_____   _____

_____   _____

_____   _____

                        Subtotal: _____

            Total grams Net Carbs: _____

Number of servings of foundation vegetables: _____

Did you take your multivitamin/mineral?   ❏ YES   ❏ NO

Your omega-3 supplement?   ❏ YES   ❏ NO

Your vitamin D supplement?   ❏ YES   ❏ NO

Number of glasses of water: _____

TODAY'S JOURNAL

How are you doing on the diet? _____

_____

_____

How do you feel? _____

_____

_____

What's working for you? _____

_____

_____

Are you experiencing any challenges and how do you plan to overcome them? _____

_____

_____

How do you feel about the changes you're making? _____

_____

_____

Did you exercise today? _____
If so, what did you do and for how long? _____

_____

_____

_____

"One extends one's limits only by extending them."
—*M. Scott Peck, MD, in* The Road Less Traveled

Date: _____

TODAY'S MEALS (including portion sizes)

Breakfast: Grams Net Carbs

_____   _____

_____   _____

_____   _____

                              Subtotal: _____

Snack:

_____   _____

Lunch:

_____   _____

_____   _____

_____   _____

_____   _____

                              Subtotal: _____

Snack:

_____   _____

Dinner:

_____   _____

_____   _____

_____   _____

_____   _____

                              Subtotal: _____

                Total grams Net Carbs: _____

Number of servings of foundation vegetables: _____

Did you take your multivitamin/mineral?   ❏ YES   ❏ NO

Your omega-3 supplement?   ❏ YES   ❏ NO

Your vitamin D supplement?   ❏ YES   ❏ NO

Number of glasses of water: _____

TODAY'S JOURNAL

How are you doing on the diet? _____

_____

How do you feel? _____

_____

What's working for you? _____

_____

Are you experiencing any challenges and how do you plan to over-
come them? _____

_____

How do you feel about the changes you're making? _____

_____

Did you exercise today? _____
If so, what did you do and for how long? _____

_____

_____

FOR A NEW YOU

HEART-PROTECTIVE FATS

All natural fats have their place on the Atkins Diet, but some
are particularly heart healthy. Monounsaturated fats found in
such foods as avocados, nuts and their butters, olives and its
oil, and high-oleic safflower oil help lower your LDL ("bad")
cholesterol. Give such foods a starring role in your meals.

Date: _____

TODAY'S MEALS (including portion sizes)

Breakfast: Grams Net Carbs

_____   _____
_____   _____
_____   _____

                              Subtotal: _____

Snack:

_____   _____

Lunch:

_____   _____
_____   _____
_____   _____
_____   _____

                              Subtotal: _____

Snack:

_____   _____

Dinner:

_____   _____
_____   _____
_____   _____
_____   _____

                              Subtotal: _____
                Total grams Net Carbs: _____

Number of servings of foundation vegetables: _____

Did you take your multivitamin/mineral?   ❏ YES   ❏ NO

Your omega-3 supplement?   ❏ YES   ❏ NO

Your vitamin D supplement?   ❏ YES   ❏ NO

Number of glasses of water: _____

TODAY'S JOURNAL

How are you doing on the diet? _____

_____

How do you feel? _____

_____

What's working for you? _____

_____

Are you experiencing any challenges and how do you plan to over-
come them? _____

_____

How do you feel about the changes you're making? _____

_____

Did you exercise today? _____
If so, what did you do and for how long? _____

_____

_____

RECENT RESEARCH

WHY TAKE A DRUG WHEN DIET CAN DO THE JOB?

When researchers at Duke University had one group of overweight or obese patients follow a low-carb diet and another
group a low-fat diet supplemented with the over-the-counter
diet drug orlistat for eleven months, individuals in both
groups lost an average of about 10 percent of their weight.
Improvements in blood sugar and lipid levels were also comparable. However, the low-carb diet provided more effective
blood pressure control than did the low-fat diet bolstered by
orlistat (marketed as Xenical and Alli). So there's really no
need to take a costly drug with unpleasant side effects to lose
weight; instead, just follow a low-carb regimen. The 2010
study was published in *Archives of Internal Medicine*.

Date: _____

TODAY'S MEALS (including portion sizes)

Breakfast: Grams Net Carbs

_____   _____

_____   _____

_____   _____

                            Subtotal: _____

Snack:

_____   _____

Lunch:

_____   _____

_____   _____

_____   _____

_____   _____

                            Subtotal: _____

Snack:

_____   _____

Dinner:

_____   _____

_____   _____

_____   _____

_____   _____

                            Subtotal: _____

                Total grams Net Carbs: _____

Number of servings of foundation vegetables: _____

Did you take your multivitamin/mineral?   ❏ YES ❏ NO

Your omega-3 supplement?   ❏ YES ❏ NO

Your vitamin D supplement?   ❏ YES ❏ NO

Number of glasses of water: _____

TODAY'S JOURNAL

How are you doing on the diet? _____

_____

How do you feel? _____

_____

What's working for you? _____

_____

Are you experiencing any challenges and how do you plan to over-
come them? _____

_____

How do you feel about the changes you're making? _____

_____

Did you exercise today? _____
If so, what did you do and for how long? _____

_____

_____

FOR A NEW YOU

WORK OUT WHILE YOU WORK

Replace the chair in your office or in front of your home com-
puter or television set with a stability ball, available online or
at sporting goods stores. Be sure to get one that's the proper
size for your height. Balancing on the ball engages your ab-
dominals and quadriceps, giving you a mini workout as it
improves your posture and reduces back strain aggravated by
sitting. Or, if you prefer, switch off between your chair and
the ball after an hour or so.

Date: _____

TODAY'S MEALS (including portion sizes)

Breakfast: Grams Net Carbs

_____   _____

_____   _____

_____   _____

                                Subtotal: _____

Snack:

_____   _____

Lunch:

_____   _____

_____   _____

_____   _____

_____   _____

                                Subtotal: _____

Snack:

_____   _____

Dinner:

_____   _____

_____   _____

_____   _____

_____   _____

                                Subtotal: _____

                 Total grams Net Carbs: _____

Number of servings of foundation vegetables: _____

Did you take your multivitamin/mineral?   ❏ YES   ❏ NO

Your omega-3 supplement?   ❏ YES   ❏ NO

Your vitamin D supplement?   ❏ YES   ❏ NO

Number of glasses of water: _____

TODAY'S JOURNAL

How are you doing on the diet? _____
_____
_____

How do you feel? _____
_____
_____

What's working for you? _____
_____
_____

Are you experiencing any challenges and how do you plan to over-
come them? _____
_____
_____

How do you feel about the changes you're making? _____
_____
_____

Did you exercise today? _____
If so, what did you do and for how long? _____
_____
_____
_____

"Never order food in excess of your body weight."

—*Erma Bombeck*

Date: _____

TODAY'S MEALS (including portion sizes)

Breakfast: Grams Net Carbs

_____ _____

_____ _____

_____ _____

Subtotal: _____

Snack:

_____

Lunch:

_____ _____

_____ _____

_____ _____

_____ _____

Subtotal: _____

Snack:

_____

Dinner:

_____ _____

_____ _____

_____ _____

_____ _____

Subtotal: _____

Total grams Net Carbs: _____

Number of servings of foundation vegetables: _____

Did you take your multivitamin/mineral?   ❑ YES ❑ NO

Your omega-3 supplement?   ❑ YES ❑ NO

Your vitamin D supplement?   ❑ YES ❑ NO

Number of glasses of water: _____

TODAY'S JOURNAL

How are you doing on the diet? _____

_____

How do you feel? _____

_____

What's working for you? _____

_____

Are you experiencing any challenges and how do you plan to over-
come them? _____

_____

How do you feel about the changes you're making? _____

_____

Did you exercise today? _____
If so, what did you do and for how long? _____

_____

_____

PRESCRIBE THE RIGHT
SALAD DRESSING

Extra-virgin olive oil always gets the lion's share of the at-
tention in salad dressings. Now it's time for vinegar to take
a bow. Acetic acid in vinegar, which makes it tart, helps
stabilize blood sugar levels after a meal, an important factor
for anyone watching their weight—or with type 2 diabetes.
Acetic acid enables some sugars and starches to pass through
your intestines without being digested, minimizing their
impact on blood sugar. You'll need 2 daily teaspoons of cider
vinegar, balsamic vinegar, or red wine vinegar for this effect.
Mix with olive oil, perhaps a little mustard, and seasonings of
your choice.

WEEK 7

By now, there's a good chance that you're in OWL (or beyond). Perhaps you're already enjoying not just tomato juice "cocktail" but also the occasional Bloody Mary or glass of wine. Life is good! And it's getting better with every week. As you broaden your food choices and add more carbs to your daily intake each week or so, it's natural for your weight loss to slow as you get closer to your goal weight. As long as you're continuing to gradually trim those pounds and inches, you're on the right track. Although we recommend that you add Phase 2 foods in the order listed on page 17, you can vary that order if you prefer. Just be sure to record what you eat and any reactions you have, and back off any food that stimulates cravings or slows your weight loss. So, you could introduce yogurt before berries, if you wish, or even a small piece of dark baking chocolate before tomato juice. The more you can personalize the program to your needs and taste preferences, the more likely you are to stay the course.

Phase: _____ Daily Net Carb Target:_____ grams

MY CURRENT STATS

Chest: _____ inches   Waist: _____ inches
Hips: _____ inches   Upper arms: _____ inches
Thighs: _____ inches   Calves: _____ inches
Weight: _____ pounds
BMI: _____   WHR: _____

How do you feel about your results over the previous week? _____
_____
_____

Did you miss any particular foods? If so, which ones? _____
_____

Did any foods provoke carb cravings, and if so, which ones? _____
_____
_____

Were you hungry between meals and/or snacks? _____
Is your energy level high, low, or medium? _____
Do your clothes fit better? _____
Have you found yourself unable to find a low-carb meal or encoun-
tered similar challenges? If so, how did you deal with it? _____
_____
_____

Would you handle this differently in the future? If so, how? _____
_____
_____

Do you plan to change the phase and/or Net Carb level this week?
_____

Do you plan to add any new foods this week? If so, which ones?
_____
_____

Do you plan to exercise this week? If so, describe: _____
_____
_____

Do you anticipate anything interfering with eating low carb this
week? If so, how do you plan to work around it? _____
_____
_____

Describe your emotions over the last week, along with other relevant feelings and thoughts. _____
_____
_____

Date: _____

TODAY'S MEALS (including portion sizes)

Breakfast: Grams Net Carbs

_____   _____

_____   _____

_____   _____

                        Subtotal: _____

Snack:

_____   _____

Lunch:

_____   _____

_____   _____

_____   _____

_____   _____

                        Subtotal: _____

Snack:

_____   _____

Dinner:

_____   _____

_____   _____

_____   _____

_____   _____

                        Subtotal: _____

            Total grams Net Carbs: _____

Number of servings of foundation vegetables: _____

Did you take your multivitamin/mineral?   ❏ YES ❏ NO

Your omega-3 supplement?   ❏ YES ❏ NO

Your vitamin D supplement?   ❏ YES ❏ NO

Number of glasses of water: _____

TODAY'S JOURNAL

How are you doing on the diet? _____

_____

How do you feel? _____

_____

What's working for you? _____

_____

Are you experiencing any challenges and how do you plan to over-come them? _____

_____

How do you feel about the changes you're making? _____

_____

Did you exercise today? _____
If so, what did you do and for how long? _____

_____

_____

RECENT RESEARCH

SATURATED FAT IS NOT THE CULPRIT

In the context of a low-carb diet, research consistently shows that saturated fat is not harmful. In one study, published in 2010 in *Lipids*, researchers at the University of Connecticut explored what happens to saturated fat levels in subjects on the Atkins Diet compared to others on a low-fat diet. Both diets contained the same number of calories, but the Atkins Diet contained three times the amount of saturated fat. Subjects on both diets lost weight; however, after twelve weeks, the Atkins dieters showed consistently greater reductions in the percentage of saturated fat in their blood. Yes, those who ate *more* saturated fat had *less* in their bloodstream than those who ate less saturated fat.

Date: _____

TODAY'S MEALS (including portion sizes)

Breakfast: Grams Net Carbs

_____ _____

_____ _____

_____ _____

Subtotal: _____

Snack:

_____ _____

Lunch:

_____ _____

_____ _____

_____ _____

_____ _____

Subtotal: _____

Snack:

_____ _____

Dinner:

_____ _____

_____ _____

_____ _____

_____ _____

Subtotal: _____

Total grams Net Carbs: _____

Number of servings of foundation vegetables: _____

Did you take your multivitamin/mineral?   ❏ YES ❏ NO

Your omega-3 supplement?   ❏ YES ❏ NO

Your vitamin D supplement?   ❏ YES ❏ NO

Number of glasses of water: _____

TODAY'S JOURNAL

How are you doing on the diet? _____

_____

How do you feel? _____

_____

What's working for you? _____

_____

Are you experiencing any challenges and how do you plan to over-
come them? _____

_____

How do you feel about the changes you're making? _____

_____

Did you exercise today? _____
If so, what did you do and for how long? _____

_____

_____

FOR A NEW YOU

EXERCISE EARLY FOR BETTER SLEEP

If you exercise early in the morning and have difficulty getting enough sleep, you might want to bunk in longer and work
out later—but not too late. Ideally, exercise at least five or six
hours before bedtime, although hatha yoga or gentle stretching is fine. Vigorous exercise raises your endorphin levels allowing you to achieve deeper sleep, but it also elevates your
core body temperature (and therefore your metabolism). Exercising at the very time of day you want to lower it in order
to stimulate the release of melatonin, the sleep hormone, is
counterproductive.

Date: _____

TODAY'S MEALS (including portion sizes)

Breakfast: Grams Net Carbs

_____   _____

_____   _____

_____   _____

Subtotal: _____

Snack:

_____   _____

Lunch:

_____   _____

_____   _____

_____   _____

_____   _____

Subtotal: _____

Snack:

_____   _____

Dinner:

_____   _____

_____   _____

_____   _____

_____   _____

Subtotal: _____

Total grams Net Carbs: _____

Number of servings of foundation vegetables: _____
Did you take your multivitamin/mineral?   ❏ YES ❏ NO
Your omega-3 supplement?   ❏ YES ❏ NO
Your vitamin D supplement?   ❏ YES ❏ NO
Number of glasses of water: _____

TODAY'S JOURNAL

How are you doing on the diet? _____

_____

_____

How do you feel? _____

_____

_____

What's working for you? _____

_____

_____

Are you experiencing any challenges and how do you plan to over-
come them? _____

_____

_____

How do you feel about the changes you're making? _____

_____

_____

Did you exercise today? _____
If so, what did you do and for how long? _____

_____

_____

_____

"When it is obvious that the goals cannot be reached, don't
adjust the goals, adjust the action steps."

—*Confucius*

Date: _____

TODAY'S MEALS (including portion sizes)

Breakfast: Grams Net Carbs

_____   _____

_____   _____

_____   _____

                              Subtotal: _____

Snack:

_____   _____

Lunch:

_____   _____

_____   _____

_____   _____

_____   _____

                              Subtotal: _____

Snack:

_____   _____

Dinner:

_____   _____

_____   _____

_____   _____

_____   _____

                              Subtotal: _____

                   Total grams Net Carbs: _____

Number of servings of foundation vegetables: _____

Did you take your multivitamin/mineral?   ❑ YES   ❑ NO

Your omega-3 supplement?   ❑ YES   ❑ NO

Your vitamin D supplement?   ❑ YES   ❑ NO

Number of glasses of water: _____

TODAY'S JOURNAL

How are you doing on the diet? _____

_____

How do you feel? _____

_____

What's working for you? _____

_____

Are you experiencing any challenges and how do you plan to overcome them? _____

_____

How do you feel about the changes you're making? _____

_____

Did you exercise today? _____
If so, what did you do and for how long? _____

_____

_____

FOR A NEW YOU

EAT YOUR CHOLESTEROL BLOCKERS

Plant stanols and sterols are lipids, substances similar to fats that help block the absorption of cholesterol (also a lipid) into your bloodstream. You'll find plenty of them in Brussels sprouts, cauliflower, broccoli, and similar veggies, another reason to be sure to get your 12–15 grams of foundation vegetables each day. Stanols and sterols are also found in nuts, seeds, olives, avocadoes, and whole grains. Locally grown, in-season vegetables in a variety of colors provide the highest levels of these two micronutrients. For maximum absorption, serve them with oil or fat.

Date: _____

TODAY'S MEALS (including portion sizes)

Breakfast: Grams Net Carbs

_____   _____

_____   _____

_____   _____

                                    Subtotal: _____

Snack:

_____   _____

Lunch:

_____   _____

_____   _____

_____   _____

_____   _____

                                    Subtotal: _____

Snack:

_____   _____

Dinner:

_____   _____

_____   _____

_____   _____

_____   _____

                                    Subtotal: _____

                        Total grams Net Carbs: _____

Number of servings of foundation vegetables: _____

Did you take your multivitamin/mineral?   ❑ YES   ❑ NO

Your omega-3 supplement?   ❑ YES   ❑ NO

Your vitamin D supplement?   ❑ YES   ❑ NO

Number of glasses of water: _____

TODAY'S JOURNAL

How are you doing on the diet? _____

_____

How do you feel? _____

_____

What's working for you? _____

_____

Are you experiencing any challenges and how do you plan to over-
come them? _____

_____

How do you feel about the changes you're making? _____

_____

Did you exercise today? _____
If so, what did you do and for how long? _____

_____

_____

SO A CALORIE ISN'T ALWAYS A CALORIE

Even though you count carbs not calories on Atkins, a 2012
study by researchers at the United States Department of
Agriculture is revealing. It concludes that the standard method
used to tally the number of calories in foods may not always be
accurate. Specifically, almonds appear to supply less energy—
and therefore fewer calories—than previously assumed. It
seems that the structure of cell walls in almonds locks in some
of the fat, making your GI tract unable to absorb it. The high
fiber content renders some of the fat indigestible, in effect
"lowering" the calories needed to burn it off. The revised calorie count for an ounce of almonds is 129 calories (down from
168–170). A previous study found similar results for pistachios.

Date: _____

TODAY'S MEALS (including portion sizes)

Breakfast: Grams Net Carbs

_____   _____

_____   _____

_____   _____

                            Subtotal: _____

Snack:

_____   _____

Lunch:

_____   _____

_____   _____

_____   _____

_____   _____

                            Subtotal: _____

Snack:

_____   _____

Dinner:

_____   _____

_____   _____

_____   _____

_____   _____

                            Subtotal: _____

                Total grams Net Carbs: _____

Number of servings of foundation vegetables: _____

Did you take your multivitamin/mineral?   ❏ YES ❏ NO

Your omega-3 supplement?   ❏ YES ❏ NO

Your vitamin D supplement?   ❏ YES ❏ NO

Number of glasses of water: _____

TODAY'S JOURNAL

How are you doing on the diet? _____

_____

How do you feel? _____

_____

What's working for you? _____

_____

Are you experiencing any challenges and how do you plan to over-come them? _____

_____

How do you feel about the changes you're making? _____

_____

Did you exercise today? _____
If so, what did you do and for how long? _____

_____

_____

FOR A NEW YOU

GET A PEDOMETER

You may have heard the recommendation to walk 10,000 steps (close to five miles) a day to achieve optimal health. But you don't have to be a "walkoholic" to slim down and improve your health. Wearing a pedometer that counts your steps as you go about your daily activities can be extremely motivating. You'll be amazed how all those trips up and down the stairs to the second floor, making dinner, walking to the bus, and up and down the halls at work add up. For more information, go to www.thewalkingsite.com/10000steps.html.

Date: _____

TODAY'S MEALS (including portion sizes)

Breakfast: Grams Net Carbs

_____   _____

_____   _____

_____   _____

Subtotal: _____

Snack:

_____   _____

Lunch:

_____   _____

_____   _____

_____   _____

_____   _____

Subtotal: _____

Snack:

_____   _____

Dinner:

_____   _____

_____   _____

_____   _____

_____   _____

Subtotal: _____

Total grams Net Carbs: _____

Number of servings of foundation vegetables: _____

Did you take your multivitamin/mineral?   ❏ YES   ❏ NO

Your omega-3 supplement?   ❏ YES   ❏ NO

Your vitamin D supplement?   ❏ YES   ❏ NO

Number of glasses of water: _____

TODAY'S JOURNAL

How are you doing on the diet? _____

_____

_____

How do you feel? _____

_____

_____

What's working for you? _____

_____

_____

Are you experiencing any challenges and how do you plan to over-
come them? _____

_____

_____

How do you feel about the changes you're making? _____

_____

_____

Did you exercise today? _____
If so, what did you do and for how long? _____

_____

_____

_____

"By prevailing over all obstacles and distractions, one may
unfailingly arrive at his chosen goal or destination."
                                    —*Christopher Columbus*

WEEK 8

You have probably found that Atkins low-carb products have made it easier for you to stay on plan, just as they're designed to do. But not all low-carb specialty foods are formulated with the same ingredients and some may provoke gastric distress. Others may prompt food cravings that you haven't experienced for weeks. The insulin response of Atkins products is carefully tested on human subjects—and the appropriate phases indicated on the packaging—but we cannot vouch for other companies' products. Always check the Nutritional Facts panel for the number of Net Carbs (subtract fiber and sugar alcohols from total carbs), as the term "low carb" doesn't conform to any set standard. That said, such convenience foods can make it easier to stay with the program regardless of where your obligations take you at mealtime or snack time. Atkins products are the perfect complement to foundation vegetables and other whole foods. Keep a few frozen Atkins entrées in your freezer and you'll always have something to eat on hand, even when there's no time to cook.

Phase: _____ Daily Net Carb Target: _____ grams

MY CURRENT STATS

Chest: _____ inches Waist: _____ inches

Hips: _____ inches Upper arms: _____ inches

Thighs: _____ inches Calves: _____ inches

Weight: _____ pounds

BMI: _____   WHR: _____

How do you feel about your results over the previous week? _____

_____

_____

Did you miss any particular foods? If so, which ones? _____

_____

_____

Did any foods provoke carb cravings, and if so, which ones? _____

_____

_____

Were you hungry between meals and/or snacks? _____

Is your energy level high, low, or medium? _____

Do your clothes fit better? _____

Have you found yourself unable to find a low-carb meal or encountered similar challenges? If so, how did you deal with it? _____

_____

_____

Would you handle this differently in the future? If so, how? _____

_____

_____

Do you plan to change phase and/or Net Carb level this week?

_____

Do you plan to add any new foods this week? If so, which ones?

_____

_____

Do you plan to exercise this week? If so, describe: _____

_____

_____

Do you anticipate anything interfering with eating low carb this
week? If so, how do you plan to work around it? _____

_____

_____

Describe your emotions over the last week, along with other relevant feelings and thoughts. _____

_____

_____

Date: _____

TODAY'S MEALS (including portion sizes)

Breakfast: Grams Net Carbs

_____   _____

_____   _____

_____   _____

                                    Subtotal: _____

Snack:

_____   _____

Lunch:

_____   _____

_____   _____

_____   _____

_____   _____

                                    Subtotal: _____

Snack:

_____   _____

Dinner:

_____   _____

_____   _____

_____   _____

_____   _____

                                    Subtotal: _____

                Total grams Net Carbs: _____

Number of servings of foundation vegetables: _____
Did you take your multivitamin/mineral?   ❏ YES   ❏ NO
Your omega-3 supplement?   ❏ YES   ❏ NO
Your vitamin D supplement?   ❏ YES   ❏ NO
Number of glasses of water: _____

TODAY'S JOURNAL

How are you doing on the diet? _____

_____

How do you feel? _____

_____

What's working for you? _____

_____

Are you experiencing any challenges and how do you plan to over-
come them? _____

_____

How do you feel about the changes you're making? _____

_____

Did you exercise today? _____
If so, what did you do and for how long? _____

_____

_____

DON'T CONFUSE THIRST WITH HUNGER

Because many of us are chronically dehydrated, our signals
can sometimes get crossed. If you've recently eaten either a
meal or a snack and still feel hungry, have a drink of water, a
cup of tea or coffee, or another carb-free beverage, wait ten
minutes, and see if your hunger has disappeared.

Date: _____

TODAY'S MEALS (including portion sizes)

Breakfast: Grams Net Carbs

_____   _____

_____   _____

_____   _____

                                 Subtotal: _____

Snack:

_____   _____

Lunch:

_____   _____

_____   _____

_____   _____

                                 Subtotal: _____

Snack:

_____   _____

Dinner:

_____   _____

_____   _____

_____   _____

_____   _____

                                 Subtotal: _____

                    Total grams Net Carbs: _____

Number of servings of foundation vegetables: _____

Did you take your multivitamin/mineral?   ❏ YES   ❏ NO

Your omega-3 supplement?   ❏ YES   ❏ NO

Your vitamin D supplement?   ❏ YES   ❏ NO

Number of glasses of water: _____

TODAY'S JOURNAL

How are you doing on the diet? _____

_____

How do you feel? _____

_____

What's working for you? _____

_____

Are you experiencing any challenges and how do you plan to over-
come them? _____

_____

How do you feel about the changes you're making? _____

_____

Did you exercise today? _____
If so, what did you do and for how long? _____

_____

_____

RECENT RESEARCH

NOT JUST WHAT BUT ALSO WHEN

In a recent study in the Netherlands, researchers fed rats
either rodent chow, chow plus saturated fat, or chow plus a
sugar solution. One group of rats could eat at will, but the
others were given either the fat or sugar water only during
their inactive period. Rats that drank all their sugar solution
in their *inactive* period gained more weight than those that
also did so during their active period, despite the total caloric
intake being the same. If these results apply to humans as
well, it appears that the worst time to consume high-sugar
snack foods is while watching television!

Date: _____

TODAY'S MEALS (including portion sizes)

Breakfast: Grams Net Carbs
_____   _____
_____   _____
_____   _____
                              Subtotal: _____
Snack:
_____   _____

Lunch:
_____   _____
_____   _____
_____   _____
_____   _____
                              Subtotal: _____
Snack:
_____   _____

Dinner:
_____   _____
_____   _____
_____   _____
_____   _____
                              Subtotal: _____
                   Total grams Net Carbs: _____

Number of servings of foundation vegetables: _____
Did you take your multivitamin/mineral?   ❏ YES ❏ NO
Your omega-3 supplement?   ❏ YES ❏ NO
Your vitamin D supplement?   ❏ YES ❏ NO
Number of glasses of water: _____

TODAY'S JOURNAL

How are you doing on the diet? _____

_____

How do you feel? _____

_____

What's working for you? _____

Are you experiencing any challenges and how do you plan to over-come them? _____

_____

How do you feel about the changes you're making? _____

_____

Did you exercise today? _____
If so, what did you do and for how long? _____

_____

_____

FOR A NEW YOU

WASTE NOT, WANT NOT

According to a 2004 study at the University of Arizona, on average, people discard as much as 25 percent of the food they purchase. To make the most of your food budget and eliminate waste, plan the week's meals, make a list, and stick to it. By avoiding impulse purchases, you'll also make it easier to exert the willpower necessary to reach your weight and health goals in a timely fashion.

Date: _____

TODAY'S MEALS (including portion sizes)

Breakfast: Grams Net Carbs

_____   _____

_____   _____

_____   _____

                              Subtotal: _____

Snack:

_____   _____

Lunch:

_____   _____

_____   _____

_____   _____

_____   _____

                              Subtotal: _____

Snack:

_____   _____

Dinner:

_____   _____

_____   _____

_____   _____

_____   _____

                              Subtotal: _____

                   Total grams Net Carbs: _____

Number of servings of foundation vegetables: _____

Did you take your multivitamin/mineral?   ❏ YES   ❏ NO

Your omega-3 supplement?   ❏ YES   ❏ NO

Your vitamin D supplement?   ❏ YES   ❏ NO

Number of glasses of water: _____

TODAY'S JOURNAL

How are you doing on the diet? _____
_____
_____

How do you feel? _____
_____
_____

What's working for you? _____
_____
_____

Are you experiencing any challenges and how do you plan to over-
come them? _____
_____
_____

How do you feel about the changes you're making? _____
_____
_____

Did you exercise today? _____
If so, what did you do and for how long? _____
_____
_____
_____

"Arriving at one goal is the starting point to another."
—*John Dewey, philosopher, psychologist, and educator*

Date: _____

TODAY'S MEALS (including portion sizes)

Breakfast: Grams Net Carbs

_____   _____

_____   _____

_____   _____

                              Subtotal: _____

Snack:

_____   _____

Lunch:

_____   _____

_____   _____

_____   _____

_____   _____

                              Subtotal: _____

Snack:

_____   _____

Dinner:

_____   _____

_____   _____

_____   _____

_____   _____

                              Subtotal: _____

               Total grams Net Carbs: _____

Number of servings of foundation vegetables: _____

Did you take your multivitamin/mineral?   ❑ YES ❑ NO

Your omega-3 supplement?   ❑ YES ❑ NO

Your vitamin D supplement?   ❑ YES ❑ NO

Number of glasses of water: _____

TODAY'S JOURNAL

How are you doing on the diet? _____

_____

How do you feel? _____

_____

What's working for you? _____

_____

Are you experiencing any challenges and how do you plan to over-
come them? _____

_____

How do you feel about the changes you're making? _____

_____

Did you exercise today? _____
If so, what did you do and for how long? _____

_____

_____

FOR A NEW YOU

FIBER-RICH BEANS

Lentils, dried peas, kidney beans, and other legumes are good
plant sources of protein and excellent sources of cholesterol-
lowering fiber. With the exception of tofu (made from soybeans), legumes are also relatively high in carbs. Once you've
reintroduced them into your diet, eat them in moderation—
sprinkled over salads, for example, or as a component in soup.
And focus on those lower in carbs, including edamame (green
soybeans), black soybeans, and split peas.

Date: _____

TODAY'S MEALS (including portion sizes)

Breakfast: Grams Net Carbs

_____   _____

_____   _____

_____   _____

Subtotal: _____

Snack:

_____   _____

Lunch:

_____   _____

_____   _____

_____   _____

_____   _____

Subtotal: _____

Snack:

_____   _____

Dinner:

_____   _____

_____   _____

_____   _____

_____   _____

Subtotal: _____

Total grams Net Carbs: _____

Number of servings of foundation vegetables: _____

Did you take your multivitamin/mineral?   ❏ YES   ❏ NO

Your omega-3 supplement?   ❏ YES   ❏ NO

Your vitamin D supplement?   ❏ YES   ❏ NO

Number of glasses of water: _____

TODAY'S JOURNAL

How are you doing on the diet? _____

_____

How do you feel? _____

_____

What's working for you? _____

_____

Are you experiencing any challenges and how do you plan to over-
come them? _____

_____

How do you feel about the changes you're making? _____

_____

Did you exercise today? _____
If so, what did you do and for how long? _____

_____

_____

RECENT RESEARCH

USE A KNIFE, EAT LESS

According to a 2012 study at the University of Arizona, cutting
your food into bite-size pieces makes it seem larger and therefore more filling than when served in one piece, despite having
identical nutritional content. Researchers presented college
students with either a whole bagel or one cut into quarters.
After twenty minutes, the students were given a meal, of
which they could eat as much as they wished, along with any
remaining bagel. The students who originally received a whole
bagel ate more of the meal and more of any leftover bagel than
did those who initially received a cut-up bagel, resulting in a
higher calorie (and carb) intake. Cut-up food appears more
satiating, making it easier to exert portion control.

Date: _____

TODAY'S MEALS (including portion sizes)

Breakfast: Grams Net Carbs

_____   _____

_____   _____

_____   _____

Subtotal: _____

Snack:

_____   _____

Lunch:

_____   _____

_____   _____

_____   _____

_____   _____

Subtotal: _____

Snack:

_____   _____

Dinner:

_____   _____

_____   _____

_____   _____

_____   _____

Subtotal: _____

Total grams Net Carbs: _____

Number of servings of foundation vegetables: _____

Did you take your multivitamin/mineral?   ❑ YES   ❑ NO

Your omega-3 supplement?   ❑ YES   ❑ NO

Your vitamin D supplement?   ❑ YES   ❑ NO

Number of glasses of water: _____

TODAY'S JOURNAL

How are you doing on the diet? _____
_____

How do you feel? _____
_____

What's working for you? _____
_____

Are you experiencing any challenges and how do you plan to over-
come them? _____
_____

How do you feel about the changes you're making? _____
_____

Did you exercise today? _____
If so, what did you do and for how long? _____
_____
_____

PAIR UP WITH AN ATKINS BUDDY

There is nothing like someone having a similar experience to
get you through rough spots, celebrate your successes, and
swap meal ideas. Ideally, team up with someone of the same
gender and a roughly similar amount of weight to lose. You
may also feel more comfortable with a person close to your
age, as weight loss becomes more challenging with passing
years. Your buddy doesn't have to live near you. With e-mail,
Skype, and cell phones, you can stay in touch regularly. Or
visit the Atkins Community where you can post a Forum
topic requesting a buddy. Strangely enough, it's sometimes
easier to talk about sensitive issues with a virtual friend.

WEEK 9

After weeks of sailing through the Atkins experience, you may have come up against a plateau—meaning that despite complying with the program, your weight hasn't budged in at least four weeks. If not, count your lucky stars and ignore this paragraph! Just to be clear, if your clothes fit better or your measurements have decreased, you're not experiencing a plateau. But if you are stuck, you may have reached your tolerance for carbs without realizing it. To remedy, try decreasing your daily intake by 10 grams of Net Carbs. If that doesn't work, go down another 5 grams. Once weight loss resumes, move up by 5-gram weekly increments. Increasing your activity level and/or omitting alcohol if you've reintroduced it may also help. Keeping a journal is actually an excellent way to diagnose the problem and get the needle on the scale moving again. Record *everything* that goes into your mouth, including lemon juice and sweeteners, and be vigilant about portion size. You may find that you're eating more than you think you are. Most important, be patient. This, too, will pass.

Phase: _____ Daily Net Carb Target: _____ grams

MY CURRENT STATS

Chest: _____ inches   Waist: _____ inches

Hips: _____ inches   Upper arms:_____ inches

Thighs: _____ inches   Calves: _____ inches

Weight: _____ pounds

BMI: _____   WHR: _____

How do you feel about your results over the previous week? _____
_____
_____

Did you miss any particular foods? If so, which ones? _____
_____
_____

Did any foods provoke carb cravings, and if so, which ones? _____
_____
_____

Were you hungry between meals and/or snacks? _____
Is your energy level high, low, or medium? _____
Do your clothes fit better? _____
Have you found yourself unable to find a low-carb meal or encoun-
tered similar challenges? If so, how did you deal with it? _____
_____
_____

Would you handle this differently in the future? If so, how? _____
_____
_____

Do you plan to change phase and/or Net Carb level this week?
_____

Do you plan to add any new foods this week? If so, which ones?
_____
_____

Do you plan to exercise this week? If so, describe: _____
_____
_____

Do you anticipate anything interfering with eating low carb this
week? If so, how do you plan to work around it? _____
_____
_____

Describe your emotions over the last week, along with other relevant feelings and thoughts. _____
_____
_____

Date: _____

TODAY'S MEALS (including portion sizes)

Breakfast: Grams Net Carbs

_____   _____
_____   _____
_____   _____

                              Subtotal: _____

Snack:

_____   _____

Lunch:

_____   _____
_____   _____
_____   _____
_____   _____

                              Subtotal: _____

Snack:

_____   _____

Dinner:

_____   _____
_____   _____
_____   _____
_____   _____

                              Subtotal: _____
                  Total grams Net Carbs: _____

Number of servings of foundation vegetables: _____

Did you take your multivitamin/mineral?   ❑ YES   ❑ NO

Your omega-3 supplement?   ❑ YES   ❑ NO

Your vitamin D supplement?   ❑ YES   ❑ NO

Number of glasses of water: _____

TODAY'S JOURNAL

How are you doing on the diet? _____
_____
_____

How do you feel? _____
_____
_____

What's working for you? _____
_____

Are you experiencing any challenges and how do you plan to over-
come them? _____
_____
_____

How do you feel about the changes you're making? _____
_____
_____

Did you exercise today? _____
If so, what did you do and for how long? _____
_____
_____
_____

"Whoever wants to reach a distant goal must take small steps."
—*novelist Saul Bellow*

Date: _____

TODAY'S MEALS (including portion sizes)

Breakfast: Grams Net Carbs

_____   _____

_____   _____

_____   _____

                            Subtotal: _____

Snack:

_____   _____

Lunch:

_____   _____

_____   _____

_____   _____

_____   _____

                            Subtotal: _____

Snack:

_____   _____

Dinner:

_____   _____

_____   _____

_____   _____

_____   _____

                            Subtotal: _____

                Total grams Net Carbs: _____

Number of servings of foundation vegetables: _____

Did you take your multivitamin/mineral?   ❏ YES   ❏ NO

Your omega-3 supplement?   ❏ YES   ❏ NO

Your vitamin D supplement?   ❏ YES   ❏ NO

Number of glasses of water: _____

TODAY'S JOURNAL

How are you doing on the diet? _____

_____

How do you feel? _____

_____

What's working for you? _____

_____

Are you experiencing any challenges and how do you plan to over-
come them? _____

_____

How do you feel about the changes you're making? _____

_____

Did you exercise today? _____
If so, what did you do and for how long? _____

_____

_____

FOR A NEW YOU

DON'T LET THESE FISH GET AWAY

Fish is an excellent source of protein and a natural component
of the Atkins Diet. Aim for two or three servings a week.
Coldwater fish, such as salmon, herring, sardines, sea trout,
bluefish, and mackerel are higher in fat than their warm-
water cousins, making them richer in heart-healthy omega-3s.
If you simply don't like fish of any sort, grass-fed beef and
wild game are a better source of omega-3s than other meats,
and walnuts and flaxseed are vegetable sources, as are blue-
green algae supplements.

Date: _____

TODAY'S MEALS (including portion sizes)

Breakfast: Grams Net Carbs

_____   _____

_____   _____

_____   _____

Subtotal: _____

Snack:

_____

Lunch:

_____   _____

_____   _____

_____   _____

_____   _____

Subtotal: _____

Snack:

_____   _____

Dinner:

_____   _____

_____   _____

_____   _____

_____   _____

Subtotal: _____

Total grams Net Carbs: _____

Number of servings of foundation vegetables: _____

Did you take your multivitamin/mineral?   ❏ YES   ❏ NO

Your omega-3 supplement?   ❏ YES   ❏ NO

Your vitamin D supplement?   ❏ YES   ❏ NO

Number of glasses of water: _____

TODAY'S JOURNAL

How are you doing on the diet? _____

_____

How do you feel? _____

_____

What's working for you? _____

_____

Are you experiencing any challenges and how do you plan to overcome them? _____

_____

How do you feel about the changes you're making? _____

_____

Did you exercise today? _____
If so, what did you do and for how long? _____

_____

_____

RECENT RESEARCH

DOCTORS OFTEN RELUCTANT TO DISCUSS WEIGHT

According to research published in 2011 in *Improving Obesity Management in Adult Primary Care*, 70 percent of obese patients are *not* diagnosed as such by their physician. And 63 percent receive no weight-loss counseling from them. How come? Now that practitioners regard their patients as customers, they don't want to make them uncomfortable by initiating such a discussion. Nor is there time in a 15–20-minute appointment to discuss this sensitive issue. Most physicians have little if any training in nutrition and don't feel qualified to treat obesity. The most effective way to get your doctor to discuss your weight is for you to raise the subject.

Date: _____

TODAY'S MEALS (including portion sizes)

Breakfast: Grams Net Carbs

_____   _____
_____   _____
_____   _____

                                    Subtotal: _____

Snack:
_____   _____

Lunch:
_____   _____
_____   _____
_____   _____
_____   _____

                                    Subtotal: _____

Snack:
_____   _____

Dinner:
_____   _____
_____   _____
_____   _____
_____   _____

                                    Subtotal: _____
                        Total grams Net Carbs: _____

Number of servings of foundation vegetables: _____

Did you take your multivitamin/mineral?   ❏ YES ❏ NO
Your omega-3 supplement?   ❏ YES ❏ NO
Your vitamin D supplement?   ❏ YES ❏ NO
Number of glasses of water: _____

TODAY'S JOURNAL

How are you doing on the diet? _____

_____

How do you feel? _____

_____

What's working for you? _____

_____

Are you experiencing any challenges and how do you plan to over-
come them? _____

_____

How do you feel about the changes you're making? _____

_____

Did you exercise today? _____
If so, what did you do and for how long? _____

_____

_____

FOR A NEW YOU

KNOW WHEN TO LEAVE THE TABLE

Don't linger at the table once you're done eating. Unless it's
Thanksgiving or you're at a dinner party, thirty minutes is
plenty of time for a meal. Otherwise, you might be tempted
to continue grazing.

Date: _____

TODAY'S MEALS (including portion sizes)

Breakfast: Grams Net Carbs

_____   _____

_____   _____

_____   _____

                              Subtotal: _____

Snack:

_____   _____

Lunch:

_____   _____

_____   _____

_____   _____

_____   _____

                              Subtotal: _____

Snack:

_____   _____

Dinner:

_____   _____

_____   _____

_____   _____

_____   _____

                              Subtotal: _____

                    Total grams Net Carbs: _____

Number of servings of foundation vegetables: _____

Did you take your multivitamin/mineral?   ❏ YES   ❏ NO

Your omega-3 supplement?   ❏ YES   ❏ NO

Your vitamin D supplement?   ❏ YES   ❏ NO

Number of glasses of water: _____

TODAY'S JOURNAL

How are you doing on the diet? _____

_____

_____

How do you feel? _____

_____

_____

What's working for you? _____

_____

_____

Are you experiencing any challenges and how do you plan to over-
come them? _____

_____

_____

How do you feel about the changes you're making? _____

_____

_____

Did you exercise today? _____
If so, what did you do and for how long? _____

_____

_____

_____

"We ought not to look back unless it is to derive useful lessons
from past errors, and for the purpose of profiting by dear bought
experience."

—*George Washington*

Date: _____

TODAY'S MEALS (including portion sizes)

Breakfast: Grams Net Carbs

_____   _____

_____   _____

_____   _____

Subtotal: _____

Snack:

_____   _____

Lunch:

_____   _____

_____   _____

_____   _____

_____   _____

Subtotal: _____

Snack:

_____   _____

Dinner:

_____   _____

_____   _____

_____   _____

_____   _____

Subtotal: _____

Total grams Net Carbs: _____

Number of servings of foundation vegetables: _____

Did you take your multivitamin/mineral?   ❑ YES   ❑ NO

Your omega-3 supplement?   ❑ YES   ❑ NO

Your vitamin D supplement?   ❑ YES   ❑ NO

Number of glasses of water: _____

TODAY'S JOURNAL

How are you doing on the diet? _____

_____

How do you feel? _____

_____

What's working for you? _____

_____

Are you experiencing any challenges and how do you plan to over-come them? _____

_____

How do you feel about the changes you're making? _____

_____

Did you exercise today? _____
If so, what did you do and for how long? _____

_____

_____

MORE THAN SKIN DIFFERENT

There are avocados, and then there are avocados. Be sure to purchase Hass avocados, which have a pebbly greenish-black skin, and are significantly lower in carbs than the larger, glossy green Florida avocados.

Date: _____

TODAY'S MEALS (including portion sizes)

Breakfast: Grams Net Carbs

_____   _____

_____   _____

_____   _____

                                        Subtotal: _____

Snack:

_____   _____

Lunch:

_____   _____

_____   _____

_____   _____

_____   _____

                                        Subtotal: _____

Snack:

_____   _____

Dinner:

_____   _____

_____   _____

_____   _____

_____   _____

                                        Subtotal: _____

                        Total grams Net Carbs: _____

Number of servings of foundation vegetables: _____

Did you take your multivitamin/mineral?   ❏ YES   ❏ NO

Your omega-3 supplement?   ❏ YES   ❏ NO

Your vitamin D supplement?   ❏ YES   ❏ NO

Number of glasses of water: _____

TODAY'S JOURNAL

How are you doing on the diet? _____

_____

How do you feel? _____

_____

What's working for you? _____

_____

Are you experiencing any challenges and how do you plan to overcome them? _____

_____

How do you feel about the changes you're making? _____

_____

Did you exercise today? _____
If so, what did you do and for how long? _____

_____

_____

RECENT RESEARCH

LOSE MORE BELLY FAT ON LOW CARB

A study from Johns Hopkins University presented in 2012 found that overweight or obese but otherwise healthy individuals who followed a low-carb weight-loss diet such as Atkins shed on average 10 more pounds over a six-month period than subjects on a low-fat diet containing the same number of calories. Researchers also found no adverse effect on heart health in the low-carb group. Both groups engaged in exercise, and heart health indicators were checked before and after the study. Both groups lost weight and abdominal fat and showed lower blood pressure; however, the low-carb group lost weight faster and experienced greater reductions in weight, BMI, waist circumference, and body fat, as well abdominal fat, a key indicator of heart health.

WEEK 10

By now, you're probably getting a handle on your personal level of carbohydrate tolerance, although you simply may not have yet reached it. Knowing the number of daily grams of Net Carbs you can consume and still continue to shed weight is key to success on Atkins. The range is enormous, anywhere from 25 to 60, or even 80 grams a day, depending upon your age, gender, height, hormonal status, and activity level. If you're presently trimming less than a pound a week from your body—which is fine after more than two months on Atkins—you're likely approaching your tolerance level. Most people find that they need to do a bit of "backing" and "forthing" to find but not overshoot that number. That's one reason you increase your daily intake in 5-gram increments every week or several weeks in OWL. It's also why you're advised to add foods one by one and in one category at a time. If introducing a certain food or category stops your weight-loss progress, back off for a few weeks before trying to reintroduce it.

Phase: _____ Daily Net Carb Target: _____ grams

MY CURRENT STATS

Chest: _____ inches Waist: _____ inches

Hips: _____ inches Upper arms: _____ inches

Thighs: _____ inches Calves: _____ inches

Weight: _____ pounds

BMI: _____. WHR: _____

How do you feel about your results over the previous week? _____

_____

_____

Did you miss any particular foods? If so, which ones? _____

_____

_____

Did any foods provoke carb cravings, and if so, which ones? _____

_____

_____

Were you hungry between meals and/or snacks? _____

Is your energy level high, low, or medium? _____

Do your clothes fit better? _____

Have you found yourself unable to find a low-carb meal or encountered similar challenges? If so, how did you deal with it? _____

_____

_____

Would you handle this differently in the future? If so, how? _____

_____

_____

Do you plan to change the phase and/or Net Carb level this week?

_____

Do you plan to add any new foods this week? If so, which ones?

_____

_____

Do you plan to exercise this week? If so, describe:_____

_____

_____

Do you anticipate anything interfering with eating low carb this
week? If so, how do you plan to work around it? _____

_____

_____

Describe your emotions over the last week, along with other relevant feelings and thoughts. _____

_____

_____

Date: _____

TODAY'S MEALS (including portion sizes)

Breakfast: Grams Net Carbs

_____   _____

_____   _____

_____   _____

Subtotal: _____

Snack:

_____   _____

Lunch:

_____   _____

_____   _____

_____   _____

_____   _____

Subtotal: _____

Snack:

_____   _____

Dinner:

_____   _____

_____   _____

_____   _____

_____   _____

Subtotal: _____

Total grams Net Carbs: _____

Number of servings of foundation vegetables: _____

Did you take your multivitamin/mineral?   ❏ YES   ❏ NO

Your omega-3 supplement?   ❏ YES   ❏ NO

Your vitamin D supplement?   ❏ YES   ❏ NO

Number of glasses of water: _____

TODAY'S JOURNAL

How are you doing on the diet? _____

_____

How do you feel? _____

_____

What's working for you? _____

_____

Are you experiencing any challenges and how do you plan to over-
come them? _____

_____

How do you feel about the changes you're making? _____

_____

Did you exercise today? _____
If so, what did you do and for how long? _____

_____

_____

FIND 120 TO 150 MINUTES

That's all the time you need each week to see the benefit of
moderately vigorous exercise, according to major health organizations. The latest thinking also indicates that even short
segments of exercise can add up to great results. This could
translate to 20–25 minutes a day six days a week, perhaps in
the form of a daily 10–15 minute morning or early-evening
walk and a 10-minute midday workout with exercise bands.

Date: _____

TODAY'S MEALS (including portion sizes)

Breakfast: Grams Net Carbs

_____   _____

_____   _____

_____   _____

Subtotal: _____

Snack:

_____   _____

Lunch:

_____   _____

_____   _____

_____   _____

_____   _____

Subtotal: _____

Snack:

_____   _____

Dinner:

_____   _____

_____   _____

_____   _____

_____   _____

Subtotal: _____

Total grams Net Carbs: _____

Number of servings of foundation vegetables: _____

Did you take your multivitamin/mineral?   ❑ YES   ❑ NO

Your omega-3 supplement?   ❑ YES   ❑ NO

Your vitamin D supplement?   ❑ YES   ❑ NO

Number of glasses of water: _____

TODAY'S JOURNAL

How are you doing on the diet? _____

_____

How do you feel? _____

_____

What's working for you? _____

_____

Are you experiencing any challenges and how do you plan to over-
come them? _____

_____

How do you feel about the changes you're making? _____

_____

Did you exercise today? _____
If so, what did you do and for how long? _____

_____

_____

"If your dog is fat, you're not getting enough exercise."

—*Anonymous*

Date: _____

TODAY'S MEALS (including portion sizes)

Breakfast: Grams Net Carbs

_____   _____
_____   _____
_____   _____

                                  Subtotal: _____

Snack:

_____   _____

Lunch:

_____   _____
_____   _____
_____   _____
_____   _____

                                  Subtotal: _____

Snack:

_____   _____

Dinner:

_____   _____
_____   _____
_____   _____
_____   _____

                                  Subtotal: _____
                Total grams Net Carbs: _____

Number of servings of foundation vegetables: _____
Did you take your multivitamin/mineral?   ❏ YES   ❏ NO
Your omega-3 supplement?   ❏ YES   ❏ NO
Your vitamin D supplement?   ❏ YES   ❏ NO
Number of glasses of water: _____

TODAY'S JOURNAL

How are you doing on the diet? _____

_____

How do you feel? _____

_____

What's working for you? _____

_____

Are you experiencing any challenges and how do you plan to over-
come them? _____

_____

How do you feel about the changes you're making? _____

_____

Did you exercise today? _____
If so, what did you do and for how long? _____

_____

_____

IT'S EASY TO EAT OUT

Dine out without stressing out. Simply order a dish prepared without carb-filled sauces, and make sure the entrée is
roasted, grilled, pan-fried, or poached instead of deep-fried.
To avoid temptation, also ask for:

- Olives or cut-up veggies in lieu of the breadbasket.
- An additional serving of vegetables instead of rice or
  potato with the entrée.
- Oil and vinegar (or lemon juice) instead of the house
  dressing.
- Berries with whipped cream for dessert.

Date: _____

TODAY'S MEALS (including portion sizes)

Breakfast: Grams Net Carbs

_____   _____

_____   _____

_____   _____

                                    Subtotal: _____

Snack:

_____   _____

Lunch:

_____   _____

_____   _____

_____   _____

_____   _____

                                    Subtotal: _____

Snack:

_____   _____

Dinner:

_____   _____

_____   _____

_____   _____

_____   _____

                                    Subtotal: _____

                        Total grams Net Carbs: _____

Number of servings of foundation vegetables: _____

Did you take your multivitamin/mineral?   ❏ YES ❏ NO

Your omega-3 supplement?   ❏ YES ❏ NO

Your vitamin D supplement?   ❏ YES ❏ NO

Number of glasses of water: _____

TODAY'S JOURNAL

How are you doing on the diet? _____

_____

How do you feel? _____

_____

What's working for you? _____

_____

Are you experiencing any challenges and how do you plan to over-
come them? _____

_____

How do you feel about the changes you're making? _____

_____

Did you exercise today? _____
If so, what did you do and for how long? _____

_____

_____

RECENT RESEARCH

AMBIANCE CAN AFFECT APPETITE

A 2012 study published in *Psychological Reports* found that
when a branch of a chain restaurant set aside a section deco-
rated like a fine restaurant, complete with mood lighting, soft
music, tablecloths, and candlelight, diners had a significantly
different culinary experience. The "fine diners" ordered the
same food as those in the conventional area of the restaurant,
but spent almost 5 percent longer at their meal and ate only
86 percent of the food on their plates rather than the 95 percent eaten by "casual diners." As a result, the fine diners ate
less, but gave the same food a higher rating on a question-
naire. The takeaway? Eat in a more relaxed environment and
you may enjoy your meals more and eat less.

Date: _____

TODAY'S MEALS (including portion sizes)

Breakfast: Grams Net Carbs

_____   _____

_____   _____

_____   _____

                                    Subtotal: _____

Snack:

_____   _____

Lunch:

_____   _____

_____   _____

_____   _____

_____   _____

                                    Subtotal: _____

Snack:

_____   _____

Dinner:

_____   _____

_____   _____

_____   _____

_____   _____

                                    Subtotal: _____

                      Total grams Net Carbs: _____

Number of servings of foundation vegetables: _____

Did you take your multivitamin/mineral?   ❏ YES ❏ NO

Your omega-3 supplement?   ❏ YES ❏ NO

Your vitamin D supplement?   ❏ YES ❏ NO

Number of glasses of water: _____

TODAY'S JOURNAL

How are you doing on the diet? _____

_____

How do you feel? _____

_____

What's working for you? _____

_____

Are you experiencing any challenges and how do you plan to overcome them? _____

_____

How do you feel about the changes you're making? _____

_____

Did you exercise today? _____
If so, what did you do and for how long? _____

_____

_____

DRESS THE PART

When exercising, be sure to wear appropriate footgear as well as comfortable clothes that allow you a full range of movement and that "breathe," so you don't get overheated or chilled, as perspiration dries. Wearing two or more layers allows you to remove and replace layers as you warm up and cool down. Of course, any old T-shirt, baggy sweatpants, and college sweatshirt would serve, but purchasing some nice exercise duds is also a good motivator to get out there and work up a sweat!

Date: _____

TODAY'S MEALS (including portion sizes)

Breakfast: Grams Net Carbs

_____   _____
_____   _____
_____   _____

                            Subtotal: _____

Snack:

_____   _____

Lunch:

_____   _____
_____   _____
_____   _____
_____   _____

                            Subtotal: _____

Snack:

_____   _____

Dinner:

_____   _____
_____   _____
_____   _____
_____   _____

                            Subtotal: _____
              Total grams Net Carbs: _____

Number of servings of foundation vegetables: _____
Did you take your multivitamin/mineral?   ❏ YES   ❏ NO
Your omega-3 supplement?   ❏ YES   ❏ NO
Your vitamin D supplement?   ❏ YES   ❏ NO
Number of glasses of water: _____

TODAY'S JOURNAL

How are you doing on the diet? _____
_____
_____

How do you feel? _____
_____
_____

What's working for you? _____
_____
_____

Are you experiencing any challenges and how do you plan to overcome them? _____
_____
_____

How do you feel about the changes you're making? _____
_____
_____

Did you exercise today? _____
If so, what did you do and for how long? _____
_____
_____
_____

"If you can imagine it, you can achieve it; if you can dream it, you can become it."

—*William Arthur Ward, author of* Fountains of Faith

Date: _____

TODAY'S MEALS (including portion sizes)

Breakfast: Grams Net Carbs

_____   _____

_____   _____

_____   _____

                            Subtotal: _____

Snack:

_____   _____

Lunch:

_____   _____

_____   _____

_____   _____

_____   _____

                            Subtotal: _____

Snack:

_____   _____

Dinner:

_____   _____

_____   _____

_____   _____

_____   _____

                            Subtotal: _____

                  Total grams Net Carbs: _____

Number of servings of foundation vegetables: _____

Did you take your multivitamin/mineral?   ❏ YES   ❏ NO

Your omega-3 supplement?   ❏ YES   ❏ NO

Your vitamin D supplement?   ❏ YES   ❏ NO

Number of glasses of water: _____

TODAY'S JOURNAL

How are you doing on the diet? _____

_____

How do you feel? _____

_____

What's working for you? _____

_____

Are you experiencing any challenges and how do you plan to over-
come them? _____

_____

How do you feel about the changes you're making? _____

_____

Did you exercise today? _____
If so, what did you do and for how long? _____

_____

_____

PICK THE BETTER SAFFLOWER

Safflower oil contains primarily polyunsaturated fat (PUFA),
meaning it's liquid both at room temperature and when re-
frigerated. Safflower oil imparts no taste to food, which can
be an advantage. However, it cannot tolerate high heat without burning, and most Americans already eat far too many
PUFAs, throwing off a preferred balance among fat types.
In high quantities, PUFAs also lower *both* HDL ("good")
and LDL ("bad") cholesterol. A better choice is high-oleic
safflower oil, which contains primarily monounsaturated
fat (MUFA), which lowers only LDL cholesterol, and has
a higher smoke point. Look for it on your supermarket's
shelves.

WEEK 11

E ven though you may be following the Atkins program to the letter, let's get real. Life happens. There may well be days when you forget to write in this journal, skip your exercise class, find yourself sharing a bag of pretzels with a buddy, or whatever. An occasional lapse is not a reason to retreat from all your good efforts. Instead of beating up on yourself for being spineless, or otherwise wallowing in guilt, simply return to the program and put past actions behind you. Another risk with such behavior is that you may be able to occasionally overdo the carbs with no immediate apparent ill effects. This could make you feel cocky about taking an occasional break from the Atkins Diet. Sooner or later, this behavior will catch up with you, and the pounds and inches you've worked so hard to eliminate will start to creep back. Do take the time to write about such an experience in this journal and consider how you can avoid similar lapses in the future.

Phase: _____ Daily Net Carb Target: _____ grams

MY CURRENT STATS
Chest: _____ inches   Waist: _____ inches
Hips: _____ inches   Upper arms: _____ inches
Thighs: _____ inches   Calves: _____ inches
Weight: _____ pounds
BMI: _____   WHR: _____

How do you feel about your results over the previous week? _____

_____

_____

Did you miss any particular foods? If so, which ones? _____

_____

_____

Did any foods provoke carb cravings, and if so, which ones? _____

_____

_____

Were you hungry between meals and/or snacks? _____

Is your energy level high, low, or medium? _____

Do your clothes fit better? _____

Have you been unable to find a low-carb meal or encountered similar challenges? If so, how did you deal with it? _____

_____

_____

Would you handle this differently in the future? If so, how? _____

_____

_____

Do you plan to change the phase and/or Net Carb level this week?

_____

Do you plan to add any new foods this week? If so, which ones?

_____

_____

Do you plan to exercise this week? If so, describe: _____

_____

_____

Do you anticipate anything interfering with eating low carb this week? If so, how do you plan to work around it? _____

_____

_____

Describe your emotions over the last week, along with other relevant feelings and thoughts. _____

_____

_____

Date: _____

TODAY'S MEALS (including portion sizes)

Breakfast: Grams Net Carbs

_____   _____

_____   _____

_____   _____

                                   Subtotal: _____

Snack:

_____   _____

Lunch:

_____   _____

_____   _____

_____   _____

_____   _____

                                   Subtotal: _____

Snack:

_____   _____

Dinner:

_____   _____

_____   _____

_____   _____

_____   _____

                                   Subtotal: _____

                      Total grams Net Carbs: _____

Number of servings of foundation vegetables: _____

Did you take your multivitamin/mineral?   ❑ YES   ❑ NO

Your omega-3 supplement?   ❑ YES   ❑ NO

Your vitamin D supplement?   ❑ YES   ❑ NO

Number of glasses of water: _____

TODAY'S JOURNAL

How are you doing on the diet? _____

_____

How do you feel? _____

_____

What's working for you? _____

_____

Are you experiencing any challenges and how do you plan to over-come them? _____

_____

How do you feel about the changes you're making? _____

_____

Did you exercise today? _____
If so, what did you do and for how long? _____

_____

_____

RECENT RESEARCH

EXERCISE MAY BENEFIT IMPULSE CONTROL

A 2011 review study conducted at Harvard University sug-gests that individuals who engage in physical exercise also eat better. But the good effects don't end there. Neurologist Miguel Alonso, one of the authors, noted, "In fact, when ex-ercise is added to a weight-loss diet, treatment of obesity is more successful and the diet is adhered to in the long run."

Date: _____

TODAY'S MEALS (including portion sizes)

Breakfast: Grams Net Carbs

_____   _____

_____   _____

_____   _____

                                                   Subtotal: _____

Snack: _____   _____

Lunch:

_____   _____

_____   _____

_____   _____

_____   _____

                                                   Subtotal: _____

Snack: _____   _____

Dinner:

_____   _____

_____   _____

_____   _____

_____   _____

                                                   Subtotal: _____

                            Total grams Net Carbs: _____

Number of servings of foundation vegetables: _____

Did you take your multivitamin/mineral?   ❑ YES   ❑ NO

Your omega-3 supplement?   ❑ YES   ❑ NO

Your vitamin D supplement?   ❑ YES   ❑ NO

Number of glasses of water: _____

TODAY'S JOURNAL

How are you doing on the diet? _____
_____

How do you feel? _____
_____

What's working for you? _____
_____

Are you experiencing any challenges and how do you plan to over-
come them? _____
_____

How do you feel about the changes you're making? _____
_____

Did you exercise today? _____
If so, what did you do and for how long? _____
_____
_____

REACH FOR THE STARS

After exercising, it's very important to spend a few minutes
stretching to help increase your flexibility and relax muscles
in order to avoid or minimize soreness from your exertions.
Stretching also helps bring your heart down to a normal rate
after vigorous physical activity. First stretch your biceps,
triceps, and hamstrings, and end with some whole-body
stretches. Be careful not to overstretch. Stretch until you feel
tension, but not pain, in the muscle group, and then hold the
stretch for twenty to thirty seconds.

Date: _____

TODAY'S MEALS (including portion sizes)

Breakfast: Grams Net Carbs

_____   _____

_____   _____

_____   _____

Subtotal: _____

Snack:

_____   _____

Lunch:

_____   _____

_____   _____

_____   _____

_____   _____

Subtotal: _____

Snack:

_____   _____

Dinner:

_____   _____

_____   _____

_____   _____

_____   _____

Subtotal: _____

Total grams Net Carbs: _____

Number of servings of foundation vegetables: _____

Did you take your multivitamin/mineral?   ❏ YES   ❏ NO

Your omega-3 supplement?   ❏ YES   ❏ NO

Your vitamin D supplement?   ❏ YES   ❏ NO

Number of glasses of water: _____

TODAY'S JOURNAL

How are you doing on the diet? _____

_____

_____

How do you feel? _____

_____

_____

What's working for you? _____

_____

_____

Are you experiencing any challenges and how do you plan to over-
come them? _____

_____

_____

How do you feel about the changes you're making? _____

_____

_____

Did you exercise today? _____
If so, what did you do and for how long? _____

_____

_____

_____

"The thing that is really hard, and really amazing, is giving up
on being perfect and beginning the work of becoming yourself."
—*author Anna Quindlen*

Date: _____

TODAY'S MEALS (including portion sizes)

Breakfast: Grams Net Carbs

_____   _____

_____   _____

_____   _____

Subtotal: _____

Snack:

_____   _____

Lunch:

_____   _____

_____   _____

_____   _____

_____   _____

Subtotal: _____

Snack:

_____   _____

Dinner:

_____   _____

_____   _____

_____   _____

_____   _____

Subtotal: _____

Total grams Net Carbs: _____

Number of servings of foundation vegetables: _____

Did you take your multivitamin/mineral?   ❏ YES ❏ NO

Your omega-3 supplement?   ❏ YES ❏ NO

Your vitamin D supplement?   ❏ YES ❏ NO

Number of glasses of water: _____

TODAY'S JOURNAL

How are you doing on the diet? _____

_____

How do you feel? _____

_____

What's working for you? _____

_____

Are you experiencing any challenges and how do you plan to over-
come them? _____

_____

How do you feel about the changes you're making? _____

_____

Did you exercise today? _____
If so, what did you do and for how long? _____

_____

_____

STEER CLEAR OF TRANS FATS

Although the Food and Drug Administration now requires
that the amount of trans fats be listed on food labels, that
doesn't mean that they have disappeared from our foods.
A loophole in the law allows foods that contain less than
0.5 grams of trans fat per serving to be marketed as *free* of
trans fats. Only the sharp-eyed customer who also checks
the list of ingredients, where they're commonly referred to as
hydrogenated or partially hydrogenated oils, will find them.
Common culprits include some shortenings as well as certain
pastries, piecrusts, cookies, crackers, and pizza dough—foods
that are not Atkins-friendly in any case.

Date: _____

TODAY'S MEALS (including portion sizes)

Breakfast: Grams Net Carbs

_____   _____

_____   _____

_____   _____

Subtotal: _____

Snack:

_____   _____

Lunch:

_____   _____

_____   _____

_____   _____

_____   _____

Subtotal: _____

Snack:

_____   _____

Dinner:

_____   _____

_____   _____

_____   _____

_____   _____

Subtotal: _____

Total grams Net Carbs: _____

Number of servings of foundation vegetables: _____

Did you take your multivitamin/mineral?   ❏ YES   ❏ NO

Your omega-3 supplement?   ❏ YES   ❏ NO

Your vitamin D supplement?   ❏ YES   ❏ NO

Number of glasses of water: _____

TODAY'S JOURNAL

How are you doing on the diet? _____

_____

How do you feel? _____

_____

What's working for you? _____

_____

Are you experiencing any challenges and how do you plan to over-
come them? _____

_____

How do you feel about the changes you're making? _____

_____

Did you exercise today? _____
If so, what did you do and for how long? _____

_____

_____

RECENT RESEARCH

VITAMIN D LEVELS
LINKED TO WEIGHT

When more than 4,600 women aged sixty-five and older were
followed for almost five years, researchers from the Kaiser
Permanente Center for Health Research found that those
with low levels of vitamin D (78 percent of all participants)
tended to be heavier to begin with and gained more weight
than did those with normal levels. Those most deficient
in vitamin D gained an average of 18.5 pounds, compared
to women with normal levels, who gained an average of
16.4 pounds. "Although it was only two pounds, over time
that can add up," study author and endocrinologist Dr. Erin
LeBlanc said in a Kaiser Permanente news release.

Date: _____

TODAY'S MEALS (including portion sizes)

Breakfast: Grams Net Carbs

_____   _____

_____   _____

_____   _____

                          Subtotal: _____

Snack:

_____   _____

Lunch:

_____   _____

_____   _____

_____   _____

_____   _____

                          Subtotal: _____

Snack:

_____   _____

Dinner:

_____   _____

_____   _____

_____   _____

_____   _____

                          Subtotal: _____

            Total grams Net Carbs: _____

Number of servings of foundation vegetables: _____

Did you take your multivitamin/mineral?   ❏ YES ❏ NO

Your omega-3 supplement?   ❏ YES ❏ NO

Your vitamin D supplement?   ❏ YES ❏ NO

Number of glasses of water: _____

TODAY'S JOURNAL

How are you doing on the diet? _____
_____

How do you feel? _____
_____

What's working for you? _____
_____

Are you experiencing any challenges and how do you plan to over-
come them? _____
_____

How do you feel about the changes you're making? _____
_____

Did you exercise today? _____
If so, what did you do and for how long? _____
_____
_____

DON'T FORGET TO BREATHE

When strength training, also known as resistance training, it's
all too easy to focus so intently on the moves themselves that
you forget to breathe. Not a good idea. Holding your breath
deprives your body of essential oxygen. (Cardio, in contrast,
makes you assume a natural breathing pattern.) Usually, you
should exhale during the part of the move that requires exer-
tion and inhale as you return to the neutral position. To get in
the habit, exaggerate your breathing and inhale through your
nose and then exhale through your mouth.

Date: _____

TODAY'S MEALS (including portion sizes)

Breakfast: Grams Net Carbs

_____   _____

_____   _____

_____   _____

                              Subtotal: _____

Snack:

_____   _____

Lunch:

_____   _____

_____   _____

_____   _____

_____   _____

                              Subtotal: _____

Snack:

_____   _____

Dinner:

_____   _____

_____   _____

_____   _____

_____   _____

                              Subtotal: _____

                  Total grams Net Carbs: _____

Number of servings of foundation vegetables: _____

Did you take your multivitamin/mineral?   ❏ YES   ❏ NO

Your omega-3 supplement?   ❏ YES   ❏ NO

Your vitamin D supplement?   ❏ YES   ❏ NO

Number of glasses of water: _____

TODAY'S JOURNAL

How are you doing on the diet? _____

_____

_____

How do you feel? _____

_____

_____

What's working for you? _____

_____

_____

Are you experiencing any challenges and how do you plan to over-
come them? _____

_____

_____

How do you feel about the changes you're making? _____

_____

_____

Did you exercise today? _____
If so, what did you do and for how long? _____

_____

_____

_____

"It is exercise alone that supports the spirits, and keeps the
mind in vigor."

—*Marcus Tullius Cicero*

WEEK 12

As you approach almost three months on Atkins, you may be zeroing in on your goal weight, especially if you didn't need to trim off too many pounds. Good work! If so, you may already have moved on to Pre-Maintenance. That is the time to proceed with caution. As you experiment with adding back the carb foods you have been avoiding since you started Atkins—including additional fruits, starchy vegetables, and whole grains—you may experience renewed carb cravings or your body's resistance to eliminating those last few pounds. Depending on your tolerance for carbs, you may not be able to reintroduce all these foods or may be able to have only occasional or small amounts of some of them. Frustrating as that experience may be, it's exactly why you add foods one at a time. By observing and recording your response to these "new" foods, you'll be getting a handle on what you will or won't be able to eat when it comes to maintaining your new shape. As long as you can sustain slow but consistent weight loss while adding these last three food categories, you'll know that you'll be able to return to eating all or most whole foods.

Phase: _____ Daily Net Carb Target: _____ grams

MY CURRENT STATS

Chest: _____ inches   Waist: _____ inches

Hips: _____ inches   Upper arms: _____ inches

Thighs: _____ inches   Calves: _____ inches

Weight: _____ pounds

BMI: _____   WHR: _____

How do you feel about your results over the previous week? _____
_____

Did you miss any particular foods? If so, which ones? _____
_____

Did any foods provoke carb cravings, and if so, which ones? _____
_____

Were you hungry between meals and/or snacks? _____

Is your energy level high, low, or medium? _____

Do your clothes fit better? _____

Have you found yourself unable to find a low-carb meal or encountered similar challenges? If so, how did you deal with it? _____
_____

Would you handle this differently in the future? If so, how? _____
_____

Do you plan to change the phase and/or Net Carb level this week?
_____

Do you plan to add any new foods this week? If so, which ones?
_____

Do you plan to exercise this week? If so, describe: _____
_____

Do you anticipate anything interfering with eating low carb this
week? If so, how do you plan to work around it? _____
_____

Describe your emotions over the last week, along with other relevant feelings and thoughts. _____
_____
_____
_____

Date: _____

TODAY'S MEALS (including portion sizes)

Breakfast: Grams Net Carbs

_____   _____
_____   _____
_____

                                   Subtotal: _____

Snack:

_____   _____

Lunch:

_____   _____
_____   _____
_____   _____
_____   _____

                                   Subtotal: _____

Snack:

_____   _____

Dinner:

_____   _____
_____   _____
_____   _____
_____   _____

                                   Subtotal: _____
                     Total grams Net Carbs: _____

Number of servings of foundation vegetables: _____
Did you take your multivitamin/mineral?   ❏ YES   ❏ NO
Your omega-3 supplement?   ❏ YES   ❏ NO
Your vitamin D supplement?   ❏ YES   ❏ NO
Number of glasses of water: _____

TODAY'S JOURNAL

How are you doing on the diet? _____

_____

How do you feel? _____

_____

What's working for you? _____

_____

Are you experiencing any challenges and how do you plan to over-
come them? _____

_____

How do you feel about the changes you're making? _____

_____

Did you exercise today? _____
If so, what did you do and for how long? _____

_____

_____

UNCOUPLE YOUR EMOTIONS
FROM FOOD

If your struggles with eating properly are entwined with
such emotional issues as feeling unloved, "different," or de-
pressed, find other ways to nurture yourself. Next time you're
tempted to soothe yourself with high-carb foods, substitute
that option with something else that will make you feel better about yourself. It could be getting a pedicure, going to a
movie with a friend, buying a new scarf, volunteering to walk
a dog at an animal shelter—which would do you both good—
or any other activity that will take you out of your head for a
while.

Date: _____

TODAY'S MEALS (including portion sizes)

Breakfast: Grams Net Carbs

_____ _____

_____ _____

_____ _____

Subtotal: _____

Snack:

_____ _____

Lunch:

_____ _____

_____ _____

_____ _____

Subtotal: _____

Snack:

_____ _____

Dinner:

_____ _____

_____ _____

_____ _____

Subtotal: _____

Total grams Net Carbs: _____

Number of servings of foundation vegetables: _____

Did you take your multivitamin/mineral?   ❑ YES ❑ NO

Your omega-3 supplement?   ❑ YES ❑ NO

Your vitamin D supplement?   ❑ YES ❑ NO

Number of glasses of water: _____

TODAY'S JOURNAL

How are you doing on the diet? _____

_____

How do you feel? _____

_____

What's working for you? _____

_____

Are you experiencing any challenges and how do you plan to overcome them? _____

_____

How do you feel about the changes you're making? _____

_____

Did you exercise today? _____
If so, what did you do and for how long? _____

_____

_____

RECENT RESEARCH

SET A GOOD EXAMPLE FOR YOUR KIDS

According to a 2011 study by researchers at both the Centers for Disease Control and Emory University, the typical teen consumes the equivalent of 28 teaspoons of added sugar a day in food and beverages. That's almost 118 grams of carbs, including but not limited to table sugar, corn syrup, and high-fructose corn syrup—three to five times more than the American Heart Association deems a "prudent upper limit." Not only are these kids almost certainly going to be overweight, they will also enter adulthood with a greater risk for heart disease and type 2 diabetes. As you change your own eating habits, your children will likely benefit as well.

Date: _____

TODAY'S MEALS (including portion sizes)

Breakfast: Grams Net Carbs

_____   _____

_____   _____

_____   _____

                            Subtotal: _____

Snack:

_____   _____

Lunch:

_____   _____

_____   _____

_____   _____

_____   _____

                            Subtotal: _____

Snack:

_____   _____

Dinner:

_____   _____

_____   _____

_____   _____

_____   _____

                            Subtotal: _____

              Total grams Net Carbs: _____

Number of servings of foundation vegetables: _____

Did you take your multivitamin/mineral?   ❑ YES   ❑ NO

Your omega-3 supplement?   ❑ YES   ❑ NO

Your vitamin D supplement?   ❑ YES   ❑ NO

Number of glasses of water: _____

TODAY'S JOURNAL

How are you doing on the diet? _____

_____

How do you feel? _____

_____

What's working for you? _____

_____

Are you experiencing any challenges and how do you plan to over-
come them? _____

_____

How do you feel about the changes you're making? _____

_____

Did you exercise today? _____
If so, what did you do and for how long? _____

_____

_____

FOR A NEW YOU

WALKING 101

Brisk walking may be a natural activity, but to get the full
fitness benefit, breathe deeply and evenly—you should be
able to carry on a conversation. Stand straight, hold your core
firm, lift your knees high, and swing your arms. Start slowly,
then speed up and slow down as needed. For the last few minutes, deliberately slow your pace to bring down your pulse.

Date: _____

TODAY'S MEALS (including portion sizes)

Breakfast: Grams Net Carbs

_____   _____

_____   _____

_____   _____

                              Subtotal: _____

Snack:

_____   _____

Lunch:

_____   _____

_____   _____

_____   _____

_____   _____

                              Subtotal: _____

Snack:

_____   _____

Dinner:

_____   _____

_____   _____

_____   _____

_____   _____

                              Subtotal: _____

            Total grams Net Carbs: _____

Number of servings of foundation vegetables: _____

Did you take your multivitamin/mineral?   ❏ YES   ❏ NO

Your omega-3 supplement?   ❏ YES   ❏ NO

Your vitamin D supplement?   ❏ YES   ❏ NO

Number of glasses of water: _____

TODAY'S JOURNAL

How are you doing on the diet? _____

_____

_____

How do you feel? _____

_____

_____

What's working for you? _____

_____

_____

Are you experiencing any challenges and how do you plan to over-
come them? _____

_____

_____

How do you feel about the changes you're making? _____

_____

_____

Did you exercise today? _____
If so, what did you do and for how long? _____

_____

_____

_____

"The capacity for hope is the most significant fact of life. It
provides human beings with a sense of destination and the
energy to get started."

—*journalist Norman Cousins*

Date: _____

TODAY'S MEALS (including portion sizes)

Breakfast: Grams Net Carbs

_____ _____

_____ _____

_____ _____

                        Subtotal: _____

Snack:

_____ _____

Lunch:

_____ _____

_____ _____

_____ _____

_____ _____

                        Subtotal: _____

Snack:

_____ _____

Dinner:

_____ _____

_____ _____

_____ _____

_____ _____

                        Subtotal: _____

        Total grams Net Carbs: _____

Number of servings of foundation vegetables: _____

Did you take your multivitamin/mineral?   ❏ YES   ❏ NO

Your omega-3 supplement?   ❏ YES   ❏ NO

Your vitamin D supplement?   ❏ YES   ❏ NO

Number of glasses of water: _____

TODAY'S JOURNAL

How are you doing on the diet? _____

_____

How do you feel? _____

_____

What's working for you? _____

_____

Are you experiencing any challenges and how do you plan to over-come them? _____

_____

How do you feel about the changes you're making? _____

_____

Did you exercise today? _____
If so, what did you do and for how long? _____

_____

_____

FOR A NEW YOU

MEATLESS MONDAYS, ANYONE?

If you are a vegetarian, are thinking of becoming one, or simply would like to reduce your consumption of animal foods, find strength in numbers. A group of more than three thousand vegetarians in the Atkins Community offers advice, support, and recipes ideas for one another. Go to www.atkins .com/Community to join.

Date: _____

TODAY'S MEALS (including portion sizes)

Breakfast: Grams Net Carbs

_____   _____

_____   _____

_____   _____

                                        Subtotal: _____

Snack:

_____   _____

Lunch:

_____   _____

_____   _____

_____   _____

_____   _____

                                        Subtotal: _____

Snack:

_____   _____

Dinner:

_____   _____

_____   _____

_____   _____

_____   _____

                                        Subtotal: _____

                          Total grams Net Carbs: _____

Number of servings of foundation vegetables: _____

Did you take your multivitamin/mineral?   ❏ YES   ❏ NO

Your omega-3 supplement?   ❏ YES   ❏ NO

Your vitamin D supplement?   ❏ YES   ❏ NO

Number of glasses of water: _____

TODAY'S JOURNAL

How are you doing on the diet? _____

_____

How do you feel? _____

_____

What's working for you? _____

_____

Are you experiencing any challenges and how do you plan to over-
come them? _____

_____

How do you feel about the changes you're making? _____

_____

Did you exercise today? _____
If so, what did you do and for how long? _____

_____

_____

RECENT RESEARCH

DON'T MIRROR BAD HABITS

Research by psychologists at the University of Birmingham
published in the *British Journal of Nutrition* shows that even
people following a weight-loss diet unconsciously mirror
the eating habits of their dining companions. To test their
theory, the researchers asked a hundred women to select from
a menu that included both healthful foods (including vegetables and fruit) and unhealthful foods (including chips and
pastries). Each study subject was paired with someone who
had previously been told to pick unhealthful options. When
the women ate with such an "unhealthy" person, they tended
to select the same unhealthful foods more often than when
eating alone or with someone making healthier choices.

Date: _____

TODAY'S MEALS (including portion sizes)

Breakfast: Grams Net Carbs

_____   _____

_____   _____

_____   _____

                              Subtotal: _____

Snack:

_____

Lunch:

_____   _____

_____   _____

_____   _____

                              Subtotal: _____

Snack:

_____

Dinner:

_____   _____

_____   _____

_____   _____

                              Subtotal: _____

                  Total grams Net Carbs: _____

Number of servings of foundation vegetables: _____

Did you take your multivitamin/mineral?   ❑ YES   ❑ NO

Your omega-3 supplement?   ❑ YES   ❑ NO

Your vitamin D supplement?   ❑ YES   ❑ NO

Number of glasses of water: _____

TODAY'S JOURNAL

How are you doing on the diet? _____

How do you feel? _____

What's working for you? _____

Are you experiencing any challenges and how do you plan to overcome them? _____

How do you feel about the changes you're making? _____

Did you exercise today? _____
If so, what did you do and for how long? _____
_____
_____

SAMPLE WORKOUT DVDS

If you're bored with your exercise routine, you may be in need of some fresh ideas. Or perhaps you feel unsure about taking a Zumba, Pilates, or tai chi class and want to get a handle on it before appearing in public. Just visit your local library, go online, or download from Netflix or another DVD rental service, all of which offer a variety of exercise programs to sample.

WEEK 13

In addition to the pleasure of seeing the change in your image in the mirror, you deserve a round of applause as you celebrate your three-month Atkins anniversary. Just as you can personalize OWL, you can do the same with Pre-Maintenance—now or when you reach that phase—meaning you can reorder the introduction of the three remaining food categories. As always, add one food at a time to see if it provokes cravings, makes you unable to stop with a small portion, or prompts weight gain. You may find it is better for you to continue to increase your Net Carb intake in 5-gram increments every week or few weeks, rather than in 10-gram increments. All this is part of the process of learning just what your body can and cannot tolerate. Also, remember that while it is fine to try to reintroduce rolled oats, quinoa, or 100 percent whole-grain bread in Pre-Maintenance, foods made from white flour and other refined grains are not recommended. If you haven't experienced a plateau in OWL, there's a good likelihood you will in Phase 3. Review the advice given on page 168 if and when weight loss plateaus.

Phase: _____ Daily Net Carb Target: _____ grams

MY CURRENT STATS

Chest: _____ inches   Waist: _____ inches

Hips: _____ inches   Upper arms: _____ inches

Thighs: _____ inches   Calves: _____ inches

Weight: _____ pounds

BMI: _____   WHR: _____

How do you feel about your results over the previous week? _____
_____
_____

Did you miss any particular foods? If so, which ones? _____
_____
_____

Did any foods provoke carb cravings, and if so, which ones? _____
_____
_____

Were you hungry between meals and/or snacks? _____
Is your energy level high, low, or medium? _____
Do your clothes fit better? _____
Have you found yourself unable to find a low-carb meal or encountered similar challenges? If so, how did you deal with it? _____
_____
_____

Would you handle this differently in the future? If so, how? _____
_____
_____

Do you plan to change the phase and/or Net Carb level this week?
_____

Do you plan to add any new foods this week? If so, which ones?
_____
_____

Do you plan to exercise this week? If so, describe: _____
_____
_____

Do you anticipate anything interfering with eating low carb this week? If so, how do you plan to work around it? _____
_____
_____

Describe your emotions over the last week, along with other relevant feelings and thoughts. _____
_____
_____

Date: _____

TODAY'S MEALS (including portion sizes)

Breakfast: Grams Net Carbs

_____   _____
_____   _____
_____   _____

                                        Subtotal: _____

Snack:

_____   _____

Lunch:

_____   _____
_____   _____
_____   _____
_____   _____

                                        Subtotal: _____

Snack:

_____   _____

Dinner:

_____   _____
_____   _____
_____   _____

                                        Subtotal: _____
                        Total grams Net Carbs: _____

Number of servings of foundation vegetables: _____
Did you take your multivitamin/mineral?   ❏ YES   ❏ NO
Your omega-3 supplement?   ❏ YES   ❏ NO
Your vitamin D supplement?   ❏ YES   ❏ NO
Number of glasses of water: _____

TODAY'S JOURNAL

How are you doing on the diet? _____

_____

_____

How do you feel? _____

_____

_____

What's working for you? _____

_____

_____

Are you experiencing any challenges and how do you plan to over-
come them? _____

_____

_____

How do you feel about the changes you're making? _____

_____

_____

Did you exercise today? _____
If so, what did you do and for how long? _____

_____

_____

_____

> "Walking is the best possible exercise. Habituate yourself to
> walk very far."
>
> —*Thomas Jefferson*

Date: _____

TODAY'S MEALS (including portion sizes)

Breakfast: Grams Net Carbs

_____   _____

_____   _____

_____   _____

                                        Subtotal: _____

Snack:

_____   _____

Lunch:

_____   _____

_____   _____

_____   _____

_____   _____

                                        Subtotal: _____

Snack:

_____   _____

Dinner:

_____   _____

_____   _____

_____   _____

_____   _____

                                        Subtotal: _____

              Total grams Net Carbs: _____

Number of servings of foundation vegetables: _____

Did you take your multivitamin/mineral?   ❏ YES   ❏ NO

Your omega-3 supplement?   ❏ YES   ❏ NO

Your vitamin D supplement?   ❏ YES   ❏ NO

Number of glasses of water: _____

TODAY'S JOURNAL

How are you doing on the diet? _____

_____

How do you feel? _____

_____

What's working for you? _____

_____

Are you experiencing any challenges and how do you plan to over-
come them? _____

_____

How do you feel about the changes you're making? _____

_____

Did you exercise today? _____
If so, what did you do and for how long? _____

_____

_____

BEWARE OF FISH "PRODUCTS"

Most fish is Atkins friendly, but some items in the seafood department are swimming in carbs. A leading brand of breaded fish sticks, for instance, logs in at more than 19 grams of Net Carbs for six sticks, and two of the same company's batter-dipped fish fillets contain 23 grams. Crab cakes are typically packed with breadcrumbs, and a 6-ounce serving of surimi, actually imitation crabmeat made from pollock and a mix of flavor enhancers and fillers, exceeds 24 grams of Net Carbs. Stay with baked, broiled, grilled, or pan-fried fish and make crab cakes without breadcrumbs or with a low-carb substitute—you'll find a recipe in the online Atkins recipe database.

Date: _____

TODAY'S MEALS (including portion sizes)

Breakfast: Grams Net Carbs

_____   _____
_____   _____
_____   _____

                              Subtotal: _____

Snack:

_____

Lunch:

_____   _____
_____   _____
_____   _____
_____   _____

                              Subtotal: _____

Snack:

_____

Dinner:

_____   _____
_____   _____
_____   _____
_____   _____

                              Subtotal: _____
              Total grams Net Carbs: _____

Number of servings of foundation vegetables: _____

Did you take your multivitamin/mineral?   ❏ YES ❏ NO

Your omega-3 supplement?   ❏ YES ❏ NO

Your vitamin D supplement?   ❏ YES ❏ NO

Number of glasses of water: _____

TODAY'S JOURNAL

How are you doing on the diet? _____

_____

How do you feel? _____

_____

What's working for you? _____

_____

Are you experiencing any challenges and how do you plan to over-
come them? _____

_____

How do you feel about the changes you're making? _____

_____

Did you exercise today? _____
If so, what did you do and for how long? _____

_____

_____

THE WRONG WAY TO SNACK

A 2011 survey of 1,007 people commissioned by Snack Facto-
ry's Pretzel Crisps reveals a disturbing trend. In lieu of three
squares a day, 40 percent of Americans would opt for eating
snack foods throughout the day. Adults younger than fifty are
more likely to display a pattern of snacking than older folks:
46 and 31 percent, respectively. Roughly 63 percent of people
are guided by tastiness rather than their waistlines when it
comes to making snack choices, and 60 percent admit to eating more than the portion size listed on the package. While
55 percent look at calories and 48 percent look at fat content,
only 31 percent look at carb content. No wonder the nation is
experiencing an obesity epidemic!

Date: _____

TODAY'S MEALS (including portion sizes)

Breakfast: Grams Net Carbs

_____   _____
_____   _____
_____   _____

                              Subtotal: _____

Snack:

_____   _____

Lunch:

_____   _____
_____   _____
_____   _____
_____   _____

                              Subtotal: _____

Snack:

_____   _____

Dinner:

_____   _____
_____   _____
_____   _____
_____   _____

                              Subtotal: _____
                Total grams Net Carbs: _____

Number of servings of foundation vegetables: _____

Did you take your multivitamin/mineral?   ❏ YES ❏ NO

Your omega-3 supplement?   ❏ YES ❏ NO

Your vitamin D supplement?   ❏ YES ❏ NO

Number of glasses of water: _____

TODAY'S JOURNAL

How are you doing on the diet? _____

_____

How do you feel? _____

_____

What's working for you? _____

_____

Are you experiencing any challenges and how do you plan to over-come them? _____

_____

How do you feel about the changes you're making? _____

_____

Did you exercise today? _____
If so, what did you do and for how long? _____

_____

_____

START SLOW TO AVOID STRAIN

Before more vigorous exercise, spend a few minutes warm-ing up. Walking will do it, as will jumping rope, marching in place, etc. Start out using just your legs and then add your arms, swinging them, raising and lowering them, crossing them in front of your chest and then extending out, or what-ever. The point is to get your heart rate up before you start more vigorous activity such as jogging or using hand weights or resistance tubes.

Date: _____

TODAY'S MEALS (including portion sizes)

Breakfast: Grams Net Carbs

_____   _____

_____   _____

_____   _____

Subtotal: _____

Snack:

_____   _____

Lunch:

_____   _____

_____   _____

_____   _____

_____   _____

Subtotal: _____

Snack:

_____   _____

Dinner:

_____   _____

_____   _____

_____   _____

_____   _____

Subtotal: _____

Total grams Net Carbs: _____

Number of servings of foundation vegetables: _____

Did you take your multivitamin/mineral?   ❏ YES   ❏ NO

Your omega-3 supplement?   ❏ YES   ❏ NO

Your vitamin D supplement?   ❏ YES   ❏ NO

Number of glasses of water: _____

TODAY'S JOURNAL

How are you doing on the diet? _____

_____

_____

How do you feel? _____

_____

_____

What's working for you? _____

_____

_____

Are you experiencing any challenges and how do you plan to over-
come them? _____

_____

_____

How do you feel about the changes you're making? _____

_____

_____

Did you exercise today? _____
If so, what did you do and for how long? _____

_____

_____

_____

"We must be willing to get rid of the life we've planned, so as to
have the life that is waiting for us."

—*author and mythologist Joseph Campbell*

Date: _____

TODAY'S MEALS (including portion sizes)

Breakfast: Grams Net Carbs

_____   _____

_____   _____

_____   _____

                                  Subtotal: _____

Snack:

_____   _____

Lunch:

_____   _____

_____   _____

_____   _____

_____   _____

                                  Subtotal: _____

Snack:

_____   _____

Dinner:

_____   _____

_____   _____

_____   _____

_____   _____

                                  Subtotal: _____

                    Total grams Net Carbs: _____

Number of servings of foundation vegetables: _____

Did you take your multivitamin/mineral?   ❏ YES ❏ NO

Your omega-3 supplement?   ❏ YES ❏ NO

Your vitamin D supplement?   ❏ YES ❏ NO

Number of glasses of water: _____

TODAY'S JOURNAL

How are you doing on the diet? _____

_____

How do you feel? _____

_____

What's working for you? _____

_____

Are you experiencing any challenges and how do you plan to over-
come them? _____

_____

How do you feel about the changes you're making? _____

_____

Did you exercise today? _____
If so, what did you do and for how long? _____

_____

_____

SHORT-CIRCUIT BINGES

Unlike a momentary lapse when you eat one high-carb food
in a moment of weakness, a binge involves gorging on high-
carb foods, particularly junk foods and sweets. If you find
yourself bingeing, obviously, the first thing is to get back on
the wagon immediately. Not tonight, not tomorrow, but right
now. Avoid any food that stimulates cravings. If you just reintroduced nuts or fruit and can't stop with an appropriate portion, stay away from them altogether. Don't eat them again
until you get things under control. If you binged on cookies
or candy, going forward an Atkins Advantage, Day Break, or
Endulge bar will give you the sweet taste you crave without
the compulsion to eat more.

Date: _____

TODAY'S MEALS (including portion sizes)

Breakfast: Grams Net Carbs

_____   _____

_____   _____

_____   _____

                                         Subtotal: _____

Snack:

_____   _____

Lunch:

_____   _____

_____   _____

_____   _____

_____   _____

                                         Subtotal: _____

Snack:

_____   _____

Dinner:

_____   _____

_____   _____

_____   _____

_____   _____

                                         Subtotal: _____

                          Total grams Net Carbs: _____

Number of servings of foundation vegetables: _____

Did you take your multivitamin/mineral?   ❏ YES   ❏ NO

Your omega-3 supplement?   ❏ YES   ❏ NO

Your vitamin D supplement?   ❏ YES   ❏ NO

Number of glasses of water: _____

TODAY'S JOURNAL

How are you doing on the diet? _____

_____

How do you feel? _____

_____

What's working for you? _____

_____

Are you experiencing any challenges and how do you plan to overcome them? _____

_____

How do you feel about the changes you're making? _____

_____

Did you exercise today? _____
If so, what did you do and for how long? _____

_____

_____

THE RIGHT CHOCOLATE

To study the results of eating certain cocoa products, researchers at the National Institute of Integrative Medicine in Melbourne, Australia, did a meta-analysis of twenty studies published over a decade, comprising a total of 856 participants. Of these, roughly half consumed 3 to 100 grams of dark chocolate or cocoa, containing 30 to 1,080 mg of flavanols daily. The other half ate low-flavanol cocoa products or none. Flavanols are plant compounds also found in green tea, berries, and red wine. The group that ate flavanols showed a small decrease in blood pressure (of 2 to 3 points)—comparable to adding regular exercise to one's lifestyle or making certain other dietary changes.

WEEK 14

Not to pry, but did you lose half a pound last week? That's good news after thirteen weeks on Atkins! You're consuming more carbs, which slows down weight loss, as it should, making this an acceptable loss at this point. If you have only 10 or fewer pounds to go you're probably in Pre-Maintenance, where you may spend a fair amount of time. It's important to understand that this phase is not the same as Lifetime Maintenance. In addition to taking you to that final phase, Pre-Maintenance is like learning to ride a bike with the aid of training wheels. Before you embark on Lifetime Maintenance, you want to be sure you have all the skills you need under your belt. This "slow and steady wins the race" approach is why you stay in Phase 3 not only until you've reached your goal weight but also until you've maintained it for four weeks. Don't race through Pre-Maintenance. The longer you "practice," the more skillful you'll be at controlling your carbs and your weight.

Phase: _____ Daily Net Carb Target: _____ grams

MY CURRENT STATS

Chest: _____ inches   Waist: _____ inches
Hips: _____ inches   Upper arms: _____ inches
Thighs: _____ inches   Calves: _____ inches
Weight: _____ pounds
BMI: _____   WHR: _____

How do you feel about your results over the previous week? _____

_____

_____

Did you miss any particular foods? If so, which ones? _____

_____

Did any foods provoke carb cravings, and if so, which ones? _____

_____

Were you hungry between meals and/or snacks? _____

Is your energy level high, low, or medium? _____

Do your clothes fit better? _____

Have you found yourself unable to find a low-carb meal or encountered similar situations? If so, how did you deal with it? _____

_____

_____

Would you handle this differently in the future? If so, how? _____

_____

Do you plan to change the phase and/or Net Carb level this week?

_____

Do you plan to add any new foods this week? If so, which ones?

_____

Do you plan to exercise this week? If so, describe: _____

_____

Do you anticipate anything interfering with eating low carb this
week? If so, how do you plan to work around it? _____

_____

_____

Describe your emotions over the last week, along with other relevant feelings and thoughts. _____

_____

_____

Date: _____

TODAY'S MEALS (including portion sizes)

Breakfast: Grams Net Carbs

_____   _____

_____   _____

_____   _____

Subtotal: _____

Snack:

_____   _____

Lunch:

_____   _____

_____   _____

_____   _____

_____   _____

Subtotal: _____

Snack:

_____   _____

Dinner:

_____   _____

_____   _____

_____   _____

_____   _____

Subtotal: _____

Total grams Net Carbs: _____

Number of servings of foundation vegetables: _____

Did you take your multivitamin/mineral?   ❑ YES   ❑ NO

Your omega-3 supplement?   ❑ YES   ❑ NO

Your vitamin D supplement?   ❑ YES   ❑ NO

Number of glasses of water: _____

TODAY'S JOURNAL

How are you doing on the diet? _____

_____

How do you feel? _____

_____

What's working for you? _____

_____

Are you experiencing any challenges and how do you plan to over-
come them? _____

_____

How do you feel about the changes you're making? _____

_____

Did you exercise today? _____
If so, what did you do and for how long? _____

_____

_____

FOR A NEW YOU

WATER TO THE RESCUE

If you find yourself dehydrated after a long walk or a workout,
particularly on a hot day, don't choose a sports drink or an
energy drink. Both are typically full of sugar or high-fructose
corn syrup. Unless you are working out vigorously for more
than an hour or participating in endurance sports, usually all
you need is plain old H_2O. And don't wait until you're done
exercising: have a few ounces of water before you begin to exercise and continue to swig as you go along in order to replace
the moisture you lose as perspiration and in your breath.

Date: _____

TODAY'S MEALS (including portion sizes)

Breakfast: Grams Net Carbs

_____   _____

_____   _____

_____   _____

                                  Subtotal: _____

Snack:

_____

Lunch:

_____   _____

_____   _____

_____   _____

_____   _____

                                  Subtotal: _____

Snack:

_____

Dinner:

_____   _____

_____   _____

_____   _____

_____   _____

                                  Subtotal: _____

                   Total grams Net Carbs: _____

Number of servings of foundation vegetables: _____

Did you take your multivitamin/mineral?   ❏ YES   ❏ NO

Your omega-3 supplement?   ❏ YES   ❏ NO

Your vitamin D supplement?   ❏ YES   ❏ NO

Number of glasses of water: _____

TODAY'S JOURNAL

How are you doing on the diet? _____
_____
_____

How do you feel? _____
_____
_____

What's working for you? _____
_____
_____

Are you experiencing any challenges and how do you plan to over-
come them? _____
_____
_____

How do you feel about the changes you're making? _____
_____
_____

Did you exercise today? _____
If so, what did you do and for how long? _____
_____
_____
_____

"Only I can change my life. No one can do it for me."
—*actress and comedienne Carol Burnett*

Date: _____

TODAY'S MEALS (including portion sizes)

Breakfast: Grams Net Carbs

_____   _____

_____   _____

_____   _____

                              Subtotal: _____

Snack:

_____   _____

Lunch:

_____   _____

_____   _____

_____   _____

_____   _____

                              Subtotal: _____

Snack:

_____   _____

Dinner:

_____   _____

_____   _____

_____   _____

_____   _____

                              Subtotal: _____

                 Total grams Net Carbs: _____

Number of servings of foundation vegetables: _____

Did you take your multivitamin/mineral?   ❏ YES   ❏ NO

Your omega-3 supplement?   ❏ YES   ❏ NO

Your vitamin D supplement?   ❏ YES   ❏ NO

Number of glasses of water: _____

TODAY'S JOURNAL

How are you doing on the diet? _____

_____

How do you feel? _____

_____

What's working for you? _____

_____

Are you experiencing any challenges and how do you plan to over-
come them? _____

_____

How do you feel about the changes you're making? _____

_____

Did you exercise today? _____
If so, what did you do and for how long? _____

_____

_____

FOR A NEW YOU

BECOME A STUDENT OF LABELS

The wide array of meat-replacement soy products includes
burgers, tempeh, and soy-based "hot dogs," "sausage," and
"meatballs." All are a boon for vegetarians—and "flexitarians"—
who are doing Atkins. However, the ingredients in these
products vary; they often include other legumes and grains—
making some more suitable than others. Don't just purchase
any veggie burger, for example. Carb counts for a single burger
can range anywhere from 2 to 15 grams of Net Carbs, so read
both the list of ingredients and the Nutritional Facts panel on
competitive products before making a purchase.

Date: _____

TODAY'S MEALS (including portion sizes)

Breakfast: Grams Net Carbs

_____   _____
_____   _____
_____   _____

                          Subtotal: _____
Snack:

_____   _____

Lunch:

_____   _____
_____   _____
_____   _____
_____   _____

                          Subtotal: _____
Snack:

_____   _____

Dinner:

_____   _____
_____   _____
_____   _____
_____   _____

                          Subtotal: _____
          Total grams Net Carbs: _____

Number of servings of foundation vegetables: _____
Did you take your multivitamin/mineral?   ❏ YES ❏ NO
Your omega-3 supplement?   ❏ YES ❏ NO
Your vitamin D supplement?   ❏ YES ❏ NO
Number of glasses of water: _____

TODAY'S JOURNAL

How are you doing on the diet? _____

_____

How do you feel? _____

_____

What's working for you? _____

_____

Are you experiencing any challenges and how do you plan to over-
come them? _____

_____

How do you feel about the changes you're making? _____

_____

Did you exercise today? _____
If so, what did you do and for how long? _____

_____

_____

RECENT RESEARCH

SUGARY SODAS CAN ALTER METABOLISM

A small 2012 study at Bangor University in Wales and published in the *European Journal of Nutrition* suggests that regular
consumption of sugary soft drinks can have negative long-term
results. Eleven people in their twenties who led moderately
active lifestyles and had not previously consumed such drinks
supplemented their regular diets with modest amounts of sugary soft drinks. After just a month, researchers found changes
in isolated muscle cells of the subjects, indicating that when
the cells identified the sugary diet, they responded by creating
an inefficient metabolism that made it harder to lose weight.
These are the same kind of adaptations found in obese people
and those with type 2 diabetes. A larger study is planned.

Date: _____

TODAY'S MEALS (including portion sizes)

Breakfast: Grams Net Carbs
_____   _____
_____   _____
_____   _____
                        Subtotal: _____
Snack:
_____   _____
Lunch:
_____   _____
_____   _____
_____   _____
                        Subtotal: _____
Snack:
_____   _____
Dinner:
_____   _____
_____   _____
_____   _____
                        Subtotal: _____
            Total grams Net Carbs: _____

Number of servings of foundation vegetables: _____
Did you take your multivitamin/mineral?   ❏ YES ❏ NO
Your omega-3 supplement?   ❏ YES ❏ NO
Your vitamin D supplement?   ❏ YES ❏ NO
Number of glasses of water: _____

TODAY'S JOURNAL

How are you doing on the diet? _____

_____

How do you feel? _____

_____

What's working for you? _____

_____

Are you experiencing any challenges and how do you plan to over-
come them? _____

_____

How do you feel about the changes you're making? _____

_____

Did you exercise today? _____
If so, what did you do and for how long? _____

_____

_____

FOR A NEW YOU

SURROUND YOURSELF WITH SUPPORTIVE PEOPLE

When you've made the decision to slim down, let your friends
and family know what you're doing and ask for their support.
Most of them will likely give it, but others may perceive your
actions as a comment on their own way of eating or weight.
Understand that their conscious or subconscious words
("You're just fine the way you are") or actions (bringing cup-
cakes to your house) are really about their own issues, not
yours. Remember, how you eat is a personal decision, as is any
lifestyle choice.

Date: _____

TODAY'S MEALS (including portion sizes)

Breakfast: Grams Net Carbs

_____   _____

_____   _____

_____   _____

                                   Subtotal: _____

Snack:

_____   _____

Lunch:

_____   _____

_____   _____

_____   _____

_____   _____

                                   Subtotal: _____

Snack:

_____   _____

Dinner:

_____   _____

_____   _____

_____   _____

_____   _____

                                   Subtotal: _____

                    Total grams Net Carbs: _____

Number of servings of foundation vegetables: _____

Did you take your multivitamin/mineral?   ❏ YES ❏ NO

Your omega-3 supplement?   ❏ YES ❏ NO

Your vitamin D supplement?   ❏ YES ❏ NO

Number of glasses of water: _____

TODAY'S JOURNAL

How are you doing on the diet? _____

_____

_____

How do you feel? _____

_____

_____

What's working for you? _____

_____

_____

Are you experiencing any challenges and how do you plan to overcome them? _____

_____

_____

How do you feel about the changes you're making? _____

_____

_____

Did you exercise today? _____

If so, what did you do and for how long? _____

_____

_____

_____

"Beautiful young people are accidents of nature, but beautiful old people are works of art."

—*Eleanor Roosevelt*

Date: _____

TODAY'S MEALS (including portion sizes)

Breakfast: Grams Net Carbs

_____   _____
_____   _____
_____   _____
                                  Subtotal: _____

Snack:

_____   _____

Lunch:

_____   _____
_____   _____
_____   _____
_____   _____
                                  Subtotal: _____

Snack:

_____   _____

Dinner:

_____   _____
_____   _____
_____   _____
_____   _____
                                  Subtotal: _____
                  Total grams Net Carbs: _____

Number of servings of foundation vegetables: _____
Did you take your multivitamin/mineral?   ❏ YES ❏ NO
Your omega-3 supplement?   ❏ YES ❏ NO
Your vitamin D supplement?   ❏ YES ❏ NO
Number of glasses of water: _____

TODAY'S JOURNAL

How are you doing on the diet? _____
_____

How do you feel? _____
_____

What's working for you? _____
_____

Are you experiencing any challenges and how do you plan to over-
come them? _____
_____

How do you feel about the changes you're making? _____
_____

Did you exercise today? _____
If so, what did you do and for how long? _____
_____
_____

CHEESE BY ANY OTHER NAME

Cheese has a place on the Atkins Diet, but if you see the words "cheese product" or "whey cheese," steer clear. Such products contain ingredients other than cheese that boost the carb count. For example, Cheez Whiz contains nineteen ingredients, starting with whey and canola oil and including sugar and "cheese culture." A 2-tablespoon serving has almost 6 grams of Net Carbs. Also avoid flavored cheeses, such as strawberry cream cheese, with more than 4 grams of Net Carbs in 2 tablespoons, almost four times that of plain cream cheese. Finally, stay away from "diet" or low-fat cheeses, which are higher in carbs than regular ones, to say nothing of being less flavorful.

WEEK 15

Sometimes we don't dare to hope for too much; other times, our hopes exceed our grasp. When you started keeping this journal, you entered the goal weight you were aiming for. Perhaps you have already reached that magic number. Or maybe you found your ambitions were overly modest and you were able to lose more than you had initially expected. Another very real possibility is that you were a bit unrealistic about what you felt was an attainable goal. Perhaps you're a woman who weighed 127 pounds the day you got married thirty years ago and were hoping to get back there. A more realistic goal might be to reach 140 pounds. Maybe you're a man whose goal was to banish 40 pounds, but with your new exercise regimen compounding the effects of doing Atkins, you've got your 32-inch waist back by losing only 35 pounds, and that's just fine. The point is to remain flexible and open to the experience. Fitting into those clothes you never thought you'd wear again is just as important as a number on the scale!

Phase: _____ Daily Net Carb Target: _____ grams

MY CURRENT STATS
Chest: _____ inches   Waist: _____ inches

Hips: _____ inches   Upper arms: _____ inches

Thighs: _____ inches   Calves: _____ inches

Weight: _____ pounds

BMI: _____   WHR: _____

How do you feel about your results over the previous week? _____
_____
_____

Did you miss any particular foods? If so, which ones? _____
_____
_____

Did any foods provoke carb cravings, and if so, which ones? _____
_____
_____

Were you hungry between meals and/or snacks? _____
Is your energy level high, low, or medium? _____
Do your clothes fit better? _____
Have you found yourself unable to find a low-carb meal or encountered similar situations? If so, how did you deal with it? _____
_____
_____

Would you handle this differently in the future? If so, how? _____
_____
_____

Do you plan to change the phase and/or Net Carb level this week?
_____

Do you plan to add any new foods this week? If so, which ones? _____
_____
_____

Do you plan to exercise this week? If so, describe: _____
_____
_____

Do you anticipate anything interfering with eating low carb this week? If so, how do you plan to work around it? _____
_____
_____

Describe your emotions over the last week, along with other relevant feelings and thoughts. _____
_____
_____

Date: _____

TODAY'S MEALS (including portion sizes)

Breakfast: Grams Net Carbs

_____   _____

_____   _____

_____   _____

                              Subtotal: _____

Snack:

_____

Lunch:

_____   _____

_____   _____

_____   _____

_____   _____

                              Subtotal: _____

Snack:

_____

Dinner:

_____   _____

_____   _____

_____   _____

_____   _____

                              Subtotal: _____

                    Total grams Net Carbs: _____

Number of servings of foundation vegetables: _____

Did you take your multivitamin/mineral?   ❏ YES   ❏ NO

Your omega-3 supplement?   ❏ YES   ❏ NO

Your vitamin D supplement?   ❏ YES   ❏ NO

Number of glasses of water: _____

TODAY'S JOURNAL

How are you doing on the diet? _____

_____

How do you feel? _____

_____

What's working for you? _____

_____

Are you experiencing any challenges and how do you plan to over-come them? _____

_____

How do you feel about the changes you're making? _____

_____

Did you exercise today? _____
If so, what did you do and for how long? _____

_____

_____

RECENT RESEARCH

LOW-CARB DIETS DON'T IMPACT KIDNEYS

One of the enduring myths about the Atkins Diet is that the amount of protein consumed could create kidney problems. However, a two-year study of more than three hundred adults (half randomly assigned to a low-carb weight-loss diet and half to a low-fat weight-loss diet) who were obese but not otherwise unhealthy, found no such evidence of harmful effects in either group. Researchers at the University of Indiana School of Medicine and other institutions found the subjects' kidneys performed their filtration role properly, with no evidence of either excess protein in the urine or fluid or electrolyte imbalances. Nor were there changes in bone density or the creation of new kidney stones.

Date: _____

TODAY'S MEALS (including portion sizes)

Breakfast: Grams Net Carbs

_____   _____

_____   _____

_____   _____

                            Subtotal: _____

Snack:

_____   _____

Lunch:

_____   _____

_____   _____

_____   _____

_____   _____

                            Subtotal: _____

Snack:

_____   _____

Dinner:

_____   _____

_____   _____

_____   _____

_____   _____

                            Subtotal: _____

                 Total grams Net Carbs: _____

Number of servings of foundation vegetables: _____

Did you take your multivitamin/mineral?   ❏ YES   ❏ NO

Your omega-3 supplement?   ❏ YES   ❏ NO

Your vitamin D supplement?   ❏ YES   ❏ NO

Number of glasses of water: _____

TODAY'S JOURNAL

How are you doing on the diet? _____
_____

How do you feel? _____
_____

What's working for you? _____
_____

Are you experiencing any challenges and how do you plan to over-
come them? _____
_____

How do you feel about the changes you're making? _____
_____

Did you exercise today? _____
If so, what did you do and for how long? _____
_____
_____

CALL IT PLAY INSTEAD

One reason that so few Americans exercise, despite knowing
how important it is to their health, is that they regard it as
work. (It's called a workout, after all!) But actually, moving
your body is the most natural form of play—think of kittens
or puppies tussling with their littermates—and one of the few
ways adults can still feel like kids again. Reset your percep-
tion of exercise and find a form that is fun for you, whether
dancing, spinning, swimming, or climbing rock walls.

Date: _____

TODAY'S MEALS (including portion sizes)

Breakfast: Grams Net Carbs

_____   _____

_____   _____

_____   _____

                                       Subtotal: _____

Snack:

_____   _____

Lunch:

_____   _____

_____   _____

_____   _____

_____   _____

                                       Subtotal: _____

Snack:

_____   _____

Dinner:

_____   _____

_____   _____

_____   _____

_____   _____

                                       Subtotal: _____

                        Total grams Net Carbs: _____

Number of servings of foundation vegetables: _____

Did you take your multivitamin/mineral?   ❏ YES   ❏ NO

Your omega-3 supplement?   ❏ YES   ❏ NO

Your vitamin D supplement?   ❏ YES   ❏ NO

Number of glasses of water: _____

TODAY'S JOURNAL

How are you doing on the diet? _____

_____

_____

How do you feel? _____

_____

_____

What's working for you? _____

_____

_____

Are you experiencing any challenges and how do you plan to over-
come them? _____

_____

_____

How do you feel about the changes you're making? _____

_____

_____

Did you exercise today? _____
If so, what did you do and for how long? _____

_____

_____

_____

"You may be disappointed if you fail, but you are doomed if you
don't try."

—opera singer Beverly Sills

Date: _____

TODAY'S MEALS (including portion sizes)

Breakfast: Grams Net Carbs

_____   _____

_____   _____

_____   _____

                    Subtotal: _____

Snack:

_____   _____

Lunch:

_____   _____

_____   _____

_____   _____

                    Subtotal: _____

Snack:

_____   _____

Dinner:

_____   _____

_____   _____

_____   _____

_____   _____

                    Subtotal: _____

           Total grams Net Carbs: _____

Number of servings of foundation vegetables: _____

Did you take your multivitamin/mineral?   ❏ YES   ❏ NO

Your omega-3 supplement?   ❏ YES   ❏ NO

Your vitamin D supplement?   ❏ YES   ❏ NO

Number of glasses of water: _____

TODAY'S JOURNAL

How are you doing on the diet? _____

_____

How do you feel? _____

_____

What's working for you? _____

_____

Are you experiencing any challenges and how do you plan to overcome them? _____

_____

How do you feel about the changes you're making? _____

_____

Did you exercise today? _____
If so, what did you do and for how long? _____

_____

_____

HAVE TEMPTATION TAMERS ON HAND

To avoid being tempted by high-carb snack foods your family or roommates may have around, be sure to have alternatives at the ready. Atkins-friendly snacks include olives, avocados, cheese, hard-boiled eggs, and after the first two weeks, nuts and seeds. Later, have berries—serve with plain whole-milk yogurt or whipped cream, perhaps—and hummus in the fridge as well.

Date: _____

TODAY'S MEALS (including portion sizes)

Breakfast: Grams Net Carbs

_____   _____

_____   _____

_____   _____

                          Subtotal: _____

Snack:

_____   _____

Lunch:

_____   _____

_____   _____

_____   _____

_____   _____

                          Subtotal: _____

Snack:

_____   _____

Dinner:

_____   _____

_____   _____

_____   _____

_____   _____

                          Subtotal: _____

              Total grams Net Carbs: _____

Number of servings of foundation vegetables: _____

Did you take your multivitamin/mineral?   ❏ YES ❏ NO

Your omega-3 supplement?   ❏ YES ❏ NO

Your vitamin D supplement?   ❏ YES ❏ NO

Number of glasses of water: _____

TODAY'S JOURNAL

How are you doing on the diet? _____

_____

How do you feel? _____

_____

What's working for you? _____

_____

Are you experiencing any challenges and how do you plan to over-
come them? _____

_____

How do you feel about the changes you're making? _____

_____

Did you exercise today? _____
If so, what did you do and for how long? _____

_____

_____

RECENT RESEARCH

GET A BIKE OR TAKE A HIKE

According to a 2010 study by Harvard researchers published
in the *Archives of Internal Medicine*, to keep your weight
constant as you move into middle age, add bicycling or brisk
walking to your daily regimen. The study looked at data
from the Nurses' Health Study II, which tracked more than
eighteen thousand women over sixteen years. The more time
the women spent cycling or walking, the more successful
they were at maintaining their weight. This suggests that it
isn't necessary to engage in vigorous exercise to stay at your
goal weight—once you reach it. In the study, the researchers
contrasted the United States with The Netherlands, where
bicycling to work is commonplace and obesity is rare.

Date: _____

TODAY'S MEALS (including portion sizes)

Breakfast: Grams Net Carbs

_____   _____

_____   _____

_____   _____

                              Subtotal: _____

Snack:

_____   _____

Lunch:

_____   _____

_____   _____

_____   _____

_____   _____

                              Subtotal: _____

Snack:

_____   _____

Dinner:

_____   _____

_____   _____

_____   _____

_____   _____

                              Subtotal: _____

                    Total grams Net Carbs: _____

Number of servings of foundation vegetables: _____

Did you take your multivitamin/mineral?   ❏ YES   ❏ NO

Your omega-3 supplement?   ❏ YES   ❏ NO

Your vitamin D supplement?   ❏ YES   ❏ NO

Number of glasses of water: _____

TODAY'S JOURNAL

How are you doing on the diet? _____
_____

How do you feel? _____
_____

What's working for you? _____
_____

Are you experiencing any challenges and how do you plan to over-
come them? _____
_____

How do you feel about the changes you're making? _____
_____

Did you exercise today? _____
If so, what did you do and for how long? _____
_____
_____

EAT BEFORE YOU GO

It's sounds counterintuitive, but if you're attending a social
function at which foods you're better off not eating will
dominate the menu, simply have your meal before you leave
home. Alternatively, have a snack first to blunt your appetite,
which should allow you to pick and choose foods carefully at
the party. This strategy can work at a buffet, but at an event
where you'll be seated at a table, simply focus on the protein
and vegetable dishes. If dessert is forced on you, have a single
bite, compliment the host, and leave the rest. There's no need
to mention your way of eating to anyone.

Date: _____

TODAY'S MEALS (including portion sizes)

Breakfast: Grams Net Carbs

_____   _____

_____   _____

_____   _____

                           Subtotal: _____

Snack:

_____   _____

Lunch:

_____   _____

_____   _____

_____   _____

_____   _____

                           Subtotal: _____

Snack:

_____   _____

Dinner:

_____   _____

_____   _____

_____   _____

_____   _____

                           Subtotal: _____

            Total grams Net Carbs: _____

Number of servings of foundation vegetables: _____

Did you take your multivitamin/mineral?   ❏ YES ❏ NO

Your omega-3 supplement?   ❏ YES ❏ NO

Your vitamin D supplement?   ❏ YES ❏ NO

Number of glasses of water: _____

TODAY'S JOURNAL

How are you doing on the diet? _____

_____

How do you feel? _____

_____

What's working for you? _____

_____

Are you experiencing any challenges and how do you plan to over-
come them? _____

_____

_____

How do you feel about the changes you're making? _____

_____

_____

Did you exercise today? _____
If so, what did you do and for how long? _____

_____

_____

_____

"People who say it cannot be done should not interrupt those
who are doing it."

—a sign at the gym where Olympic winner
and runner Michael Johnson worked out

WEEK 16

Can you believe it? You've reached the last week of this workbook, been following Atkins for almost four months, and deserve a gold star for commitment. Whether you've reached your goal weight or are still losing, there's no reason to stop tracking your carb intake and making your journal entries. As you reach or transition to a permanent way of eating that will allow you to control your weight permanently, it's important to continue your good habits. Compared to sustaining weight loss, losing weight is easy. The key, obviously, is not to revert to your old way of eating. Long after you've filled every page in this journal, continue to weigh and measure yourself weekly. As long as you know the number of daily grams of Net Carbs you can consume while keeping your weight constant, you have the tool you need to stay slim for a lifetime. Never let yourself gain more than 5 pounds, and if you do see your weight increase, act immediately by dropping 10–20 grams below your usual level of tolerance; you should be able to banish those excess pounds quickly. Then slowly increase your carb intake to return to your usual carb level. Understand that as you get older, perhaps become less active due to an injury or a new job, or experience hormonal changes, your tolerance for carbs may change and you'll need to adjust your intake level. Remember, as long as you stay with Atkins, you'll remain in control.

Phase: _____ Daily Net Carb Target: _____ grams

MY CURRENT STATS

Chest: _____ inches Waist: _____ inches

Hips: _____ inches Upper arms: _____ inches

Thighs: _____ inches Calves: _____ inches

Weight: _____ pounds

BMI: _____ WHR: _____

How do you feel about your results over the previous week? _____

Did you miss any particular foods? If so, which ones? _____

Did any foods provoke carb cravings, and if so, which ones? _____

Were you hungry between meals and/or snacks? _____

Is your energy level high, low, or medium? _____

Do your clothes fit better? _____

Have you found yourself unable to find a low-carb meal or encountered similar situations? If so, how did you deal with it? _____

Would you handle this differently in the future? If so, how? _____

Do you plan to change the phase and/or Net Carb level this week?

Do you plan to add any new foods this week? If so, which ones?

Do you plan to exercise this week? If so, describe: _____

Do you anticipate anything interfering with eating low carb this week? If so, how do you plan to work around it? _____

Describe your emotions over the last week, along with other relevant feelings and thoughts. _____

Date: _____

TODAY'S MEALS (including portion sizes)

Breakfast: Grams Net Carbs

_____   _____

_____   _____

_____   _____

                                          Subtotal: _____

Snack:

_____   _____

Lunch:

_____   _____

_____   _____

_____   _____

_____   _____

                                          Subtotal: _____

Snack:

_____   _____

Dinner:

_____   _____

_____   _____

_____   _____

_____   _____

                                          Subtotal: _____

                        Total grams Net Carbs: _____

Number of servings of foundation vegetables: _____

Did you take your multivitamin/mineral?   ❑ YES ❑ NO

Your omega-3 supplement?   ❑ YES ❑ NO

Your vitamin D supplement?   ❑ YES ❑ NO

Number of glasses of water: _____

TODAY'S JOURNAL

How are you doing on the diet? _____

_____

How do you feel? _____

_____

What's working for you? _____

_____

Are you experiencing any challenges and how do you plan to over-
come them? _____

_____

How do you feel about the changes you're making? _____

_____

Did you exercise today? _____
If so, what did you do and for how long? _____

_____

_____

REDEFINING COMFORT FOODS

When you're stressed, your body may crave carbs. Maybe it's
chocolate pudding, brownies, or a candy bar. Or perhaps it's
mashed potatoes, fries, or mac and cheese. While stress is a
given, you can retrain your brain to be satisfied with lower-
carb comfort foods instead of higher-carb ones. If sweet stuff
soothes your jangled nerves, how about sugar-free versions of
hot chocolate or chocolate macaroons, or an Atkins Endulge
bar? If savory items calm the savage beast, mashed cauliflower
mimics the texture of spuds and jicama (or in later phases
sweet potato) makes great fries. Whatever your go-to comfort
food, try to come up with a reasonable substitute.

Date: _____

TODAY'S MEALS (including portion sizes)

Breakfast: Grams Net Carbs

_____   _____

_____   _____

_____   _____

Subtotal: _____

Snack:

_____   _____

Lunch:

_____   _____

_____   _____

_____   _____

_____   _____

Subtotal: _____

Snack:

_____   _____

Dinner:

_____   _____

_____   _____

_____   _____

_____   _____

Subtotal: _____

Total grams Net Carbs: _____

Number of servings of foundation vegetables: _____

Did you take your multivitamin/mineral?   ❏ YES   ❏ NO

Your omega-3 supplement?   ❏ YES   ❏ NO

Your vitamin D supplement?   ❏ YES   ❏ NO

Number of glasses of water: _____

TODAY'S JOURNAL

How are you doing on the diet? _____

_____

How do you feel? _____

_____

What's working for you? _____

_____

Are you experiencing any challenges and how do you plan to over-
come them? _____

_____

How do you feel about the changes you're making? _____

_____

Did you exercise today? _____
If so, what did you do and for how long? _____

_____

_____

YES, DIET SODAS CAN PILE ON THE POUNDS

Drinking diet soda appears to be linked to weight gain, specifically abdominal weight gain, according to a study by researchers at the University of Texas Health Science Center at San Antonio. Of 474 participants followed for ten years, people who said they drank two or more diet sodas a day were six times more likely to see their waistline increase than those who did not drink such beverages. Abdominal obesity is associated with a number of serious health problems, including type 2 diabetes. According to Helen P. Hazuda, one of the authors, "They [the beverages] may be free of calories, but not of consequences."

Date: _____

TODAY'S MEALS (including portion sizes)

Breakfast: Grams Net Carbs

_____   _____

_____   _____

_____   _____

                              Subtotal: _____

Snack:

_____   _____

Lunch:

_____   _____

_____   _____

_____   _____

_____   _____

                              Subtotal: _____

Snack:

_____   _____

Dinner:

_____   _____

_____   _____

_____   _____

_____   _____

                              Subtotal: _____

                  Total grams Net Carbs: _____

Number of servings of foundation vegetables: _____

Did you take your multivitamin/mineral?   ❏ YES   ❏ NO

Your omega-3 supplement?   ❏ YES   ❏ NO

Your vitamin D supplement?   ❏ YES   ❏ NO

Number of glasses of water: _____

TODAY'S JOURNAL

How are you doing on the diet? _____

_____

How do you feel? _____

_____

What's working for you? _____

_____

Are you experiencing any challenges and how do you plan to over-
come them? _____

_____

How do you feel about the changes you're making? _____

_____

Did you exercise today? _____
If so, what did you do and for how long? _____

_____

_____

FOR A NEW YOU

DON'T CALL YOURSELF BAD NAMES

You can cheat on a test, your taxes, or your partner but not
with food. Eating food is neither illegal nor unprincipled, and
in any case, you're not deceiving anyone but yourself. Get it
into your head that overindulging isn't a matter of cheating
and you're not a bad person for eating certain foods. Instead,
think of your occasional fallings off the wagon as a choice.
And, yes, you might have made a poor choice yesterday if you
ate half a plate of brownies, but you can make good choices
today. Using terms such as "cheating" and "bad" perpetuates
feelings of guilt and low self-esteem that only lead to punish-
ing yourself with more bad choices.

Date: _____

TODAY'S MEALS (including portion sizes)

Breakfast: Grams Net Carbs

_____   _____

_____   _____

_____   _____

                              Subtotal: _____

Snack:

_____   _____

Lunch:

_____   _____

_____   _____

_____   _____

_____   _____

                              Subtotal: _____

Snack:

_____   _____

Dinner:

_____   _____

_____   _____

_____   _____

_____   _____

                              Subtotal: _____

                   Total grams Net Carbs: _____

Number of servings of foundation vegetables: _____

Did you take your multivitamin/mineral?   ❏ YES ❏ NO

Your omega-3 supplement?   ❏ YES ❏ NO

Your vitamin D supplement?   ❏ YES ❏ NO

Number of glasses of water: _____

TODAY'S JOURNAL

How are you doing on the diet? _____

_____

_____

How do you feel? _____

_____

_____

What's working for you? _____

_____

_____

Are you experiencing any challenges and how do you plan to over-
come them? _____

_____

_____

How do you feel about the changes you're making? _____

_____

_____

Did you exercise today? _____
If so, what did you do and for how long? _____

_____

_____

_____

> "Success is to be measured not so much by the position that one
> has reached in life as by the obstacles which he has overcome
> while trying to succeed."
>
> —*former slave, author, and presidential advisor Booker T. Washington*

Date: _____

TODAY'S MEALS (including portion sizes)

Breakfast: Grams Net Carbs

_____   _____

_____   _____

_____   _____

                                    Subtotal: _____

Snack:

_____   _____

Lunch:

_____   _____

_____   _____

_____   _____

_____   _____

                                    Subtotal: _____

Snack:

_____   _____

Dinner:

_____   _____

_____   _____

_____   _____

_____   _____

                                    Subtotal: _____

                       Total grams Net Carbs: _____

Number of servings of foundation vegetables: _____

Did you take your multivitamin/mineral?   ❑ YES   ❑ NO

Your omega-3 supplement?   ❑ YES   ❑ NO

Your vitamin D supplement?   ❑ YES   ❑ NO

Number of glasses of water: _____

TODAY'S JOURNAL

How are you doing on the diet? _____

_____

How do you feel? _____

_____

What's working for you? _____

_____

Are you experiencing any challenges and how do you plan to overcome them? _____

_____

How do you feel about the changes you're making? _____

_____

Did you exercise today? _____
If so, what did you do and for how long? _____

_____

_____

DE-STRESS FOR WEIGHT LOSS

The stress hormone cortisol and the fat-storing hormone insulin have a close relationship that bodes poorly for your health and weight. Cortisol stimulates the release of insulin. And the more fat you store, particularly around your waist, the more insulin your body produces, creating a vicious cycle. To help break this pattern, reduce your stress level with low-intensity exercise like yoga, stretching, or tai chi as well as meditation or biofeedback.

Date: _____

TODAY'S MEALS (including portion sizes)

Breakfast: Grams Net Carbs

_____   _____

_____   _____

_____   _____

Subtotal: _____

Snack:

_____   _____

Lunch:

_____   _____

_____   _____

_____   _____

_____   _____

Subtotal: _____

Snack:

_____   _____

Dinner:

_____   _____

_____   _____

_____   _____

_____   _____

Subtotal: _____

Total grams Net Carbs: _____

Number of servings of foundation vegetables: _____

Did you take your multivitamin/mineral?   ❏ YES   ❏ NO

Your omega-3 supplement?   ❏ YES   ❏ NO

Your vitamin D supplement?   ❏ YES   ❏ NO

Number of glasses of water: _____

TODAY'S JOURNAL

How are you doing on the diet? _____

_____

How do you feel? _____

_____

What's working for you? _____

_____

Are you experiencing any challenges and how do you plan to over-
come them? _____

_____

How do you feel about the changes you're making? _____

_____

Did you exercise today? _____
If so, what did you do and for how long? _____

_____

_____

RECENT RESEARCH

VITAMIN D MAY STOP THE
DEVELOPMENT OF DIABETES

A 2012 observational study published in *Diabetes Care* suggests that vitamin D supplements may help prevent type 2
diabetes in people who are at risk for the disease. The more
than two thousand study subjects were people with pre-
diabetes who were enrolled in the Diabetes Prevention Program at Tufts Medical Center. Individuals with the highest
blood serum levels of vitamin D were almost 30 percent less
likely to develop diabetes than people with the lowest levels
of the vitamin.

Date: _____

TODAY'S MEALS (including portion sizes)

Breakfast: Grams Net Carbs

_____   _____

_____   _____

_____   _____

                              Subtotal: _____

Snack:

_____   _____

Lunch:

_____   _____

_____   _____

_____   _____

_____   _____

                              Subtotal: _____

Snack:

_____   _____

Dinner:

_____   _____

_____   _____

_____   _____

_____   _____

                              Subtotal: _____

                    Total grams Net Carbs: _____

Number of servings of foundation vegetables: _____

Did you take your multivitamin/mineral?   ❏ YES ❏ NO

Your omega-3 supplement?   ❏ YES ❏ NO

Your vitamin D supplement?   ❏ YES ❏ NO

Number of glasses of water: _____

TODAY'S JOURNAL

How are you doing on the diet? _____

_____

How do you feel? _____

_____

What's working for you? _____

_____

Are you experiencing any challenges and how do you plan to over-
come them? _____

_____

How do you feel about the changes you're making? _____

_____

Did you exercise today? _____
If so, what did you do and for how long? _____

_____

_____

FOR A NEW YOU

STAY WITH IT

Once you've achieved your goal weight and begun to see
other positive changes in your life, resist the drift back to old
habits. Learn to recognize unproductive thoughts or behav-
iors as soon as they surface, and come up with techniques
to ignore or transform them. You spent months working to
achieve your goal and the last thing you want to do is undo all
that good work!

A NEW YOU

Place your "after" photo here.

The "new" me after 16 weeks
on the new Atkins Diet!

Congratulations on your life-changing achievements! You've changed not just your body, but also your habits, over the last four months, meaning you should be able to make both changes permanent. Rather than an end, this is just a "way station" on your continuing journey to maintain your new weight— or, if you still have pounds and inches to banish—achieve it. Review your journal regularly to remind yourself of what you are capable of. And if you ever find yourself tempted to revert to some old, unproductive habits, just check out your initial stats and "before" photo and compare them to where you are today!

MY CURRENT STATS

Chest: _____ inches Waist: _____ inches

Hips: _____ inches Upper arms: _____ inches

Thighs: _____ inches Calves: _____ inches

Weight: _____ pounds Dress Size/Pant Size: _____

BMI (see page 8) _____ WHR (see page 9) _____

Enter your current blood pressure and any other health statistics your physician may have provided you with. _____

_____

_____

_____

CARB COUNTER

The majority of foods on the following list are suitable for two or more phases of Atkins. To ascertain whether a particular food is acceptable for the phase you're in, see "Climbing the Carb Ladder" on page 16. When purchasing processed foods, check the Nutrition Facts label and list of ingredients. To calculate Net Carbs, subtract fiber (and sugar alcohols, if included) from grams of total carbs. Atkins Nutritionals products appear on pages 322 to 324. For a more complete list, including many processed foods, see the Carb Counter on www.atkins.com/Free-Tools.aspx. There is also an Atkins phone app for on-the-go carb counting, which you can find at www.atkins.com. To avoid confusion with acceptable products, a few products that are *not* recommended for people following the Atkins Diet are also listed.

CARB COUNTER FOOD LIST

FOOD	PORTION	NET CARBS (G)	COMMENTS
FISH			
Anchovies, canned in oil	6 ounces	0	
Anchovies, baked, grilled, pan-fried	6 ounces	0	Not breaded or batter fried
Bass, baked, grilled, pan-fried	6 ounces	0	Not breaded or batter fried
Bluefish, baked, grilled, pan-fried	6 ounces	0	Not breaded or batter fried
Catfish, baked, grilled, pan-fried	6 ounces	0	Not breaded or batter fried
Cod, baked, grilled, pan-fried	6 ounces	0	Not breaded or batter fried
Cod, dried, salted	3 ounces	0	
Eel, baked, grilled, pan-fried	6 ounces	0	Not breaded or batter fried
Fish sticks	6 pieces	18–27	Not recommended
Gefilte fish without added sugar	1 piece	2	
Grouper, baked, grilled, pan-fried	6 ounces	0	Not breaded or batter fried
Haddock, baked, grilled, pan-fried	6 ounces	0	Not breaded or batter fried
Haddock, smoked	6 ounces	0	
Halibut, baked, grilled, pan-fried	6 ounces	0	Not breaded or batter fried
Herring, baked, grilled, pan-fried	6 ounces	0	Not breaded or batter fried
Herring in sour cream	¼ cup	8	Contains added sugar
Herring, pickled	¼ cup	3.4	Many brands contain sugar
Mackerel, baked, grilled, pan-fried	6 ounces	0	Not breaded or batter fried
Mahimahi, baked, grilled, pan-fried	6 ounces	0	Not breaded or batter fried
Perch, baked, grilled, pan-fried	6 ounces	0	Not breaded or batter fried

FOOD	PORTION	NET CARBS (G)	COMMENTS
Salmon, canned	6 ounces	0	
Salmon, poached, baked, grilled, pan-fried	6 ounces	0	Not breaded or batter fried
Salmon, lox	6 ounces	0	
Salmon, smoked	6 ounces	0	
Sardines, baked, grilled, pan-fried	6 ounces	0	Not breaded or batter fried
Sardines, canned in mustard sauce	6 ounces	0	
Sardines, canned in tomato sauce	6 ounces	0.8	
Sardines, canned in oil	6 ounces	0	
Sardines, smoked	6 ounces	0	
Scrod, baked, grilled, pan-fried	6 ounces	0	Not breaded or batter fried
Shad, baked, grilled, pan-fried	6 ounces	0	Not breaded or batter fried
Sole, poached, baked, grilled, pan-fried	6 ounces	0	Not breaded or batter fried
Striped bass, baked, grilled, pan-fried	6 ounces	0	Not breaded or batter fried
Swordfish, baked, grilled, pan-fried	6 ounces	0	Not breaded or batter fried
Tilapia, baked, grilled, pan-fried	6 ounces	0	Not breaded or batter fried
Trout, baked, grilled, pan-fried	6 ounces	0	Not breaded or batter fried
Tuna, canned in oil or water	6 ounces	0	
Tuna, baked, grilled, pan-fried	6 ounces	0	Not breaded or batter fried
Trout, smoked	6 ounces	0	
SHELLFISH			
Clams, canned, drained	6 ounces	10	
Clams	6 ounces	8.7	Not breaded or batter fried
Crabmeat, fresh or canned, drained	6 ounces	0	
Crab, baked, grilled, pan-fried	6 ounces	0	Not breaded or batter fried

THE NEW ATKINS FOR A NEW YOU WORKBOOK

FOOD	PORTION	NET CARBS (G)	COMMENTS
Imitation crabmeat/surimi	6 ounces	24.7	Not recommended; contains fillers
Crawfish, steamed, grilled, pan-fried	6 ounces	0	Not breaded or batter fried
Lobster meat, boiled, steamed, grilled	6 ounces	0	
Mussels, smoked, canned in oil	6 ounces	7.5	
Mussels, steamed	6 ounces	12.6	
Octopus/calamari, steamed, pan-fried	6 ounces	6.4	Not breaded or batter fried
Oysters, canned	6 ounces	6.7	
Oysters, Eastern, steamed, baked, grilled, pan-fried	6 ounces	9.3	Not breaded or batter fried
Oysters, Pacific, steamed, baked, grilled, pan-fried	6 ounces	16.8	Not breaded or batter fried
Oysters, smoked	6 ounces	6	
Scallops, poached, baked, pan-fried	6 ounces	10.1	Not breaded or batter fried
Shrimp/prawns, steamed, baked	6 ounces	2.6	Breaded or batter fried
Squid, steamed, baked, grilled, pan-fried	6 ounces	6.4	Not breaded or batter fried
POULTRY			
Capon, baked, roasted	6 ounces		Not stuffed
Chicken, all cuts, grilled, pan-fried, poached, baked, roasted	6 ounces	0	Skin on or off; not breaded, batter fried, or stuffed
Chicken sausage, plain	1 sausage	1	Many brands contain fillers full of carbs
Duck, all cuts, grilled, pan-fried, baked, roasted	6 ounces	0	Breaded, batter fried, or stuffed
Goose, roasted	6 ounces	0	Not stuffed
Rock Cornish hen, grilled, baked, roasted	6 ounces	0	Not stuffed
Turkey, all cuts, roasted, baked, grilled, pan-fried	6 ounces	0	Not breaded, batter fried, or stuffed

FOOD	PORTION	NET CARBS (G)	COMMENTS
Turkey sausage, plain	2 ounces	0	
Turkey breakfast sausage	1 link	0.4	
MEAT			
Bacon, slab	3 slices	0.5	
Beef, any cut	6 ounces	0	
Beef jerky	1 ounce	2.6	Cured with sugar
Bologna, beef	3 slices	2.1	Contains fillers
Bologna, beef and pork	3 slices	2.2	Contains fillers
Breakfast sausage, pork	1 link	0	
Calf liver	6 ounces	8.8	
Canadian bacon	3 slices	1.4	Cured with sugar
Chorizo	2 ounces	1.1	
Corned beef	6 ounces	0.8	
Frankfurter, beef	1 frank	1.8	Contains fillers
Frankfurter, beef and pork	one 3-ounce frank	3.7	Contains fillers
Frankfurter, Hebrew National	1 frank	1	
Frankfurter, pork	1 frank	0.1	
Goat, any cut	6 ounces	0	
Ham	6 ounces	0	
Ham, deli sliced	6 ounces	3	Contains sugars
Kielbasa, beef	2 ounces	1.6	Contains fillers
Lamb, any cut	6 ounces	0	
Liverwurst	6 ounces	5.8	Contains fillers; not recommended
Olive loaf	3 ounces	5.9	Contains fillers; not recommended
Pancetta	1 ounce	0	
Pastrami, beef	6 ounces	0.6	
Pepperoni	5 pieces	0	
Pork, uncured any cut	6 ounces	0	
Pork and beef sausage	1 piece	1.1	Contains fillers
Pork sausage	3 ounces	0	
Prosciutto	6 ounces	0.5	
Roast beef, deli style	6 ounces	3	

FOOD	PORTION	NET CARBS (G)	COMMENTS
Salami, beef	3 slices	1.5	
Salami, beef and pork	3 slices	1	
Salami, pork	3 slices	0.5	
Sausage, Italian	2 ounces	0.9	Contains fillers
Spam	2 ounces	1.7	Contains fillers
Veal, any cut	6 ounces	0	
VEGETARIAN/VEGAN PROTEIN SOURCES	(SEE ALSO OTHER DAIRY PRODUCTS AND SUBSTITUTES)		
Seitan	1 piece	2	Check individual products for carb counts
Quorn burger	1	4	
Quorn roast	4 ounces	4	
Quorn unbreaded cutlet	1	3	Avoid breaded cutlets
Shirataki soy noodles	½ cup	2	
Soy "cheese"	1 slice	1	
Soy "cheese"	1 ounce	0	
Tempeh, soy	4 ounces	2	Avoid products with rice and other grains
Tofu, firm	4 ounces	1.7	
Tofu, regular	4 ounces	1.8	
Tofu, silken, firm	4 ounces	2.7	
Tofu, silken, soft	½ cup	3.2	
Tofu "bacon"	2 strips	3.3	
Tofu "Canadian bacon"	3 slices	1	
Tofu "hot dog"	1 dog	2–5	Carb counts vary by brand, depending on ingredients
Tofu bulk "sausage"	2 ounces	3	
Tofu "link sausage"	2 links	4	
Vegan "cheese," no casein	1 slice	5	
Vegan "cheese," no casein	1 ounce	6	
Veggie burger	1 burger	2	Some brands are much higher; check Nutritional Facts panel
Veggie crumbles	¾ cup	2.2	
Veggie "meatballs"	4–5 balls or 4 ounces	3.9	

FOOD	PORTION	NET CARBS (G)	COMMENTS
EGGS AND CHEESE			
Egg, large, any style	1 egg	0.4	
American cheese	1 slice or ⅔ ounces	1.5	
American cheese "food"	1 slice or ⅔ ounces	1.5	
Blue cheese, crumbled	2 tbsp.	0.4	
Boursin	2 tbsp.	1	
Brie	1 ounce	0.1	
Camembert	1 ounce	0.1	
Cheddar	1 ounce	0.4	
Cheez Whiz	2 tbsp.	5.6	Cheese product; not recommended
Cottage cheese, 2% fat	½ cup	4.1	
Cottage cheese, creamed, 4% fat	½ cup	6	
Cream cheese, chive and onion	2 tbsp.	2	
Cream cheese, plain	2 tbsp.	1.2	
Cream cheese, strawberry	2 tbsp.	4.4	Not recommended; contains added sugar
Edam	1 ounce	0.4	
Feta	1 ounce	1.2	
Fontina	1 ounce	0.4	
Goat, soft	1 ounce	0.3	
Gorgonzola	1 ounce	1.1	
Gouda	1 ounce	0.6	
Havarti	1 ounce	0	
Jarlsberg	1 ounce	1.2	
Laughing Cow	1 wedge	1	
Mascarpone	1 ounce	0	
Mozzarella, part skim	1 ounce	0.8	
Mozzarella, whole milk	1 ounce	0.6	
Muenster	1 ounce	0.3	
Neufchâtel	2 tbsp.	1	
Parmesan, chunk	1 ounce	0.9	
Parmesan, grated	1 tbsp.	0.2	

THE NEW ATKINS FOR A NEW YOU WORKBOOK

FOOD	PORTION	NET CARBS (G)	COMMENTS
Port wine spread	2 tbsp.	3	Cheese product; not recommended
Provolone	1 ounce	0.6	
Ricotta, part skim	¼ cup	3.2	
Ricotta, whole milk	¼ cup	1.9	
Romano, chunk	1 ounce	1	
Romano, grated	1 tbsp.	0	
Swiss	1 ounce	1.5	
Swiss Knight	1 wedge	0	
Velveeta	1 ounce	2.8	Cheese product; not recommended
OTHER DAIRY PRODUCTS AND SUBSTITUTES			
Almond milk, plain, unsweetened	1 cup	1	
Almond milk, vanilla, unsweetened	1 cup	1	
Butter, stick or whipped	1 tbsp.	0	
Buttermilk, cultured from 1% fat milk	1 cup	13	
Buttermilk, cultured from low-fat milk	1 cup	11.7	
Coconut milk beverage, plain, unsweetened	1 cup	1	
Coffee-mate, plain	1 tbsp.	6	Not recommended
Coffee-mate, fat-free Hazelnut	1 tbsp.	5	Not recommended
Cream, light	1 tbsp.	0.6	
Cream, heavy, liquid	1 tbsp.	0.4	
Cream, heavy, whipped	2 tbsp.	0.2	
Half-and-half	1 tbsp.	0.7	
Milk, sweetened, condensed, canned	2 tbsp.	20.8	Not recommended; contains added sugar
Milk, evaporated, 2% fat	2 tbsp.	3	
Milk, evaporated, whole	2 tbsp.	3.2	
Milk, reduced fat (2%)	1 cup	11.7	
Milk, low fat	1 cup	12.2	
Milk, nonfat/skim	1 cup	12.2	
Milk, whole	1 cup	11.7	
Rice milk, plain	1 cup	25	Not recommended; contains added sugar

FOOD	PORTION	NET CARBS (G)	COMMENTS
Rice milk, vanilla	1 cup	28	Not recommended; contains added sugar
Sour cream, light	2 tbsp.	2.2	
Sour cream, regular	2 tbsp.	0.7	
Soy milk, plain, unsweetened	1 cup	2	
Yogurt, plain unsweetened, whole milk	4 ounces	5.3	
Yogurt, Greek, plain, unsweetened, whole milk	4 ounces	3.5	
Yogurt, FAGE Total Classic Greek Yogurt, plain, whole milk	7 ounces	6.1	
VEGETABLES			
Alfalfa sprouts, raw	½ cup	0	
Artichoke, medium, steamed	1	4	
Artichoke hearts, canned	1	1	
Artichoke hearts, frozen	½ cup	2.7	
Artichoke hearts, marinated	4 pieces	4	
Arugula, raw	1 cup	0.4	
Asparagus, steamed	6 spears	1.9	
Asparagus, canned	4 spears	0.7	
Asparagus, frozen, steamed	½ cup	0.3	
Avocado, Hass	half	1.3	
Avocado, Florida	half	3.6	
Bamboo shoots, sliced, canned	½ cup	1	
Beans, fava, steamed	½ cup	12.1	
Beans, green, raw	½ cup	2.1	
Beans, green/string, steamed	½ cup	2.9	
Beans, yellow wax, steamed	½ cup	2.9	
Beet greens, steamed	½ cup	1.8	
Beets, steamed, sliced	½ cup	6.8	
Beets, canned, drained	½ cup	4.3	
Bok choy (pak choy), raw	½ cup	0.3	
Bok choy (pak choy), steamed	½ cup	0.4	
Broccoflower, steamed	½ cup	1.3	
Broccoli florets, raw	½ cup	0.8	

FOOD	PORTION	NET CARBS (G)	COMMENTS
Broccoli, frozen, chopped, steamed	½ cup	2.2	
Broccoli florets, fresh, steamed	½ cup	1.8	
Broccoli rabe, raw, chopped	½ cup	0.1	
Broccoli rabe, steamed	½ cup	0.8	
Broccolini, fresh. steamed	½ cup	1.9	
Brussels sprouts, steamed	½ cup	3.5	
Burdock, steamed	½ cup	12.1	
Cabbage, green, raw, shredded	½ cup	1.1	
Cabbage, Chinese, raw, shredded	½ cup	0.4	
Cabbage, red, raw, shredded	½ cup	1.8	
Cabbage, green, steamed, shredded	½ cup	2.7	
Cabbage, red, steamed	½ cup	3.3	
Cabbage, Savoy, steamed	½ cup	1.9	
Cardoon, steamed	½ cup	2.1	
Carrot, 7.5 inches long, raw	1	4.1	
Carrot, sliced, steamed	½ cup	4.1	
Cassava (yuca), mashed	½ cup	25.1	
Cauliflower, steamed	½ cup	1.7	
Cauliflower florets, raw	½ cup	1.6	
Celery, raw	1 stalk	1	
Celery, steamed	½ cup	1.8	
Celery root (celeriac), raw, grated	½ cup	5.8	
Celery root (celeriac), steamed	½ cup	3.6	
Chard, Swiss, steamed	½ cup	1.8	
Chayote, steamed	½ cup	1.8	
Chicory greens, steamed	½ cup	0.1	
Collard greens, steamed	1 cup	2	
Coleslaw with dressing	½ cup	6.6	Contains added sugar
Corn, canned	½ cup	14.9	
Corn, canned, cream style	½ cup	21.7	
Corn, kernels	½ cup	12.6	
Corn on the cob	1 medium	19.6	
Cucumber, sliced	½ cup	1.6	
Daikon radish, raw, sliced	½ cup	1	

FOOD	PORTION	NET CARBS (G)	COMMENTS
Dandelion greens, steamed	½ cup	1.8	
Eggplant, Italian, Chinese, Japanese, broiled	½ cup	2.3	
Endive, raw	½ cup	0.1	
Escarole, raw, chopped	½ cup	0.1	
Escarole, steamed	½ cup	0.1	
Fennel, raw	½ cup	1.8	
Fennel, braised	½ cup	1.5	
Garlic	1 clove	0.9	
Greens/salad greens, mixed, raw	1 cup	1.3	
Herbs, fresh	1 tbsp.	0–0.4	
Jerusalem artichoke, raw	½ cup	11.9	
Jicama, raw, chopped	½ cup	2.6	
Kale, steamed	½ cup	2.4	
Kohlrabi, steamed	½ cup	4.6	
Leeks, chopped	½ cup	5.5	
Lettuce, Boston or bibb, raw, chopped	1 cup	0.6	
Lettuce, iceberg, raw, shredded	1 cup	1.3	
Lettuce, loose leaf, raw	1 cup	1	
Lettuce, Romaine, raw, shredded	1 cup	0.6	
Mesclun, raw	1 cup	0.5	
Mung bean sprouts, raw	½ cup	2.2	
Mushrooms, button, fresh, raw, sliced	½ cup	0.8	
Mushrooms, button, cooked	¼ cup	2.4	
Mushrooms, Portobello, cooked	4 ounces	2.6	
Mushrooms, shiitake, cooked, sliced	¼ cup	1	
Mushrooms, straw, canned	½ cup	2	
Mustard greens, steamed	½ cup	0.1	
Nopales (cactus pads), cooked	½ cup	1	
Okra, cooked	½ cup	1.8	
Olives, black	5	0.7	
Olives, green	5	0.1	
Onion, white, raw, chopped	2 tbsp.	1.5	
Onion, white, raw, chopped	½ cup	6.1	

FOOD	PORTION	NET CARBS (G)	COMMENTS
Onions, chopped, cooked	¼ cup	4.3	
Palm, hearts of, canned	1 heart	0.7	
Parsnips, steamed	½ cup	10.2	
Peas, fresh, shelled	½ cup	6.8	
Peas, frozen	½ cup	7	
Peppers, bell, green, chopped, cooked	¼ cup	1.6	
Peppers, bell, green, chopped, raw	½ cup	2.2	
Peppers, bell, red, chopped, cooked	¼ cup	1.6	
Peppers, bell, red, chopped, raw	½ cup	3	
Potato, baked with skin	½ small	13.1	
Potato, steamed, diced	½ cup	14.2	
Potato, steamed, mashed	½ cup	13.4	
Pumpkin, cooked	½ cup	4.7	
Pumpkin, canned	½ cup	6.4	
Radicchio, raw	½ cup	0.7	
Radishes, raw	10	1.6	
Rhubarb, raw, unsweetened, diced	½ cup	1.7	
Rutabaga, steamed	½ cup	5.9	
Sauerkraut, drained	½ cup	1.2	
Scallions, raw, chopped	½ cup	2.4	
Shallots, raw, chopped	2 tbsp.	3.4	
Shallots, raw, chopped	½ cup	13.4	
Snow peas, snap peas in pod, fresh, chopped	½ cup	2.4	
Snow peas, snap peas in pod, steamed from frozen	4 ounces	2.7	
Sorrel greens, steamed	2 ounces	0.2	
Spaghetti squash, baked	½ cup	3.9	
Spinach, raw, chopped	1 cup	0.4	
Spinach, fresh, steamed	½ cup	1.2	
Spinach, frozen, steamed	½ cup	1	
Squash, acorn, baked, cubed	½ cup	10.4	
Squash, acorn, baked, mashed	½ cup	7.6	
Squash, butternut, baked, cubed	½ cup	7.5	

FOOD	PORTION	NET CARBS (G)	COMMENTS
Squash, butternut, steamed, mashed	½ cup	8.5	
Squash, Hubbard, steamed, mashed	½ cup	4.2	
Squash, summer/yellow, raw, sliced	½ cup	1.3	
Squash, summer/yellow, sliced, steamed	½ cup	2.6	
Sweet potato, baked	½ medium	9.9	
Sweet potato, steamed, cubed	½ cup	14.3	
Sweet potato, candied	½ cup	28.9	
Sweet potato, steamed, mashed	½ cup	17.4	
Taro, cooked, mashed	½ cup	19.5	
Taro leaves, steamed	½ cup	1.5	
Tomatillo, fresh, chopped	½ cup	2.6	
Tomato, cherry	10	4.6	
Tomato, plum	1	1.7	
Tomato, small	1	2.5	
Tomato, cooked	¼ cup	4.3	
Tomato, sun-dried, in oil	5 pieces	2.6	
Tomato, canned, diced, in juice	¼ cup	2	
Tomato paste, canned	2 tbsp.	4.9	
Tomato purée	2 tbsp.	2.2	
Tomatoes, canned, diced	½ cup	4	
Tomato sauce	¼ cup	4.9	Varies by product; choose one without added sugar
Tomatoes, canned, stewed	½ cup	6.6	
Turnip greens, frozen, cooked	½ cup	1.3	
Turnip greens, raw, steamed	½ cup	0.6	
Turnips, white, steamed, cubed	½ cup	2.4	
Turnips, white, steamed, mashed	½ cup	3.5	
Water chestnuts, sliced, canned	¼ cup	3.4	
Watercress, raw, chopped	½ cup	0.1	
Yams, canned, mashed	½ cup	24.6	
Yams, sliced, cooked	½ cup	16.1	
Yautía (arracache), sliced, cooked	3 ounces	26.2	
Yuca (cassava), raw	½ cup	37.4	

THE NEW ATKINS FOR A NEW YOU WORKBOOK

FOOD	PORTION	NET CARBS (G)	COMMENTS
Zucchini, raw, chopped	½ cup	1.4	
Zucchini, sliced, steamed	½ cup	1.5	
FATS, OILS, AND SALAD DRESSINGS			
Butter	1 tbsp.	0	
Margarine, hard	1 tbsp.	0.1	Not recommended
Margarine, soft/whipped	1 tbsp.	0.2	Not recommended
Canola oil	2 tbsp.	0	
Coconut oil	2 tbsp.	0	
Corn oil	2 tbsp.	0	Not recommended
Flaxseed oil	2 tbsp.	0	Do not heat
Grape seed oil	2 tbsp.	0	
Olive oil	2 tbsp.	0	
Peanut oil	2 tbsp.	0	Not recommended
Safflower oil	2 tbsp.	0	Use high-oleic type instead
Safflower oil, high oleic	2 tbsp.	0	
Sesame oil	2 tbsp.	0	Do not heat
Soybean oil	2 tbsp.	0	Not recommended
Vegetable oil	2 tbsp.	0	Not recommended
Walnut oil	2 tbsp.	0	Do not heat
Lard	2 tbsp.	0	
Vegetable shortening (Crisco)	2 tbsp.	0	Not recommended
Mayonnaise (sugar free)	1 tbsp.	0	Use brands made with canola or olive oil, not soybean or safflower oil
Miracle Whip	1 tbsp.	4	Not recommended; contains sugar, cornstarch and soybean oil
Miracle Whip Light	1 tbsp.	2.3	Not recommended; contains sugar, high-fructose corn syrup, cornstarch, and soybean oil

FOOD	PORTION	NET CARBS (G)	COMMENTS
Salad dressing, balsamic vinegar	2 tbsp.	4	Approximate; look for brands without sugar
Salad dressing, blue cheese	2 tbsp.	1.3	Approximate; look for brands without sugar
Salad dressing, Caesar	2 tbsp.	0.8	Approximate; look for brands without sugar
Salad dressing, French	2 tbsp.	5	Not recommended; too high in carbs
Salad dressing, Italian	2 tbsp.	3.1	Approximate; look for brands without sugar
Salad dressing, Ranch	2 tbsp.	1.8	Approximate; look for brands without sugar
Salad dressing, Thousand Island	2 tbsp.	4.5	
Salad dressing, vinaigrette	2 tbsp.	1	Approximate; look for brands without sugar
NON-CALORIC SWEETENERS			
Equal	1 packet	1	
Splenda	1 packet	1	
Splenda	1 tbsp.	1.5	
Stevia (Truvia, SweetLeaf)	1 packet	1	
Sugar Twin	1 packet	1	
Sweet 'N Low	1 packet	1	
Xylitol	1 tbsp.	0	
CONDIMENTS, HERBS, AND SPICES			
Anchovy paste	1 tbsp.	0	
Basil, fresh, chopped	1 tbsp.	0	
Basil, dried	1 tbsp.	0.2	
Black bean sauce	1 tsp.	0.5	
Capers	1 tbsp.	0.1	
Caponata	2 tbsp.	0	

FOOD	PORTION	NET CARBS (G)	COMMENTS
Chili peppers, ancho	1 pepper	5.1	
Chili peppers, hot cherry, fresh	½ ounce	1	
Chili peppers, hot cherry, canned	1 pepper	2.8	
Chili peppers, jalapeño, fresh, sliced	½ cup	1.7	
Chili peppers, jalapeño, pickled, canned, sliced	1 ounce	0.5	
Chili peppers, ancho, dried	1 pepper	5.1	
Chili peppers, cayenne, red, roasted, canned	1 pepper	5	
Chili powder	1 tbsp.	0	
Chili pepper, pasilla	1 pepper	1.7	
Chili pepper, serrano, sliced	½ cup	1.8	
Chipotle en adobo	2 peppers	2	
Chives, fresh, chopped	1 tbsp.	0.1	
Cilantro, fresh, chopped	1 tbsp.	0	
Clam juice	1 cup	0.2	
Coconut milk, unsweetened	½ cup	1.9	
Cocoa powder, unsweetened	1 tbsp.	1.3	
Cumin seed, dried, ground	1 tsp.	0.1	
Dill, fresh, chopped	1 tbsp.	0	
Enchilada sauce	¼ cup	4	
Fish sauce	1 tsp.	0.2	
Garlic	1 clove	0.9	
Ginger root, fresh, grated	1 tbsp.	1	
Herbs, dried (oregano, thyme, etc.)	1 tbsp.	0.8	
Hoisin sauce, no added sugar (Steel's)	2 tbsp.	1	
Horseradish, prepared	1 tbsp.	0.4	
Ketchup	1 tbsp.	3.7	Contains added sugar
Ketchup, no added sugar (Steel's)	1 tbsp.	1	
Miso paste, mellow brown	1 tbsp.	0	
Mustard, Chinese	1 tsp.	0.2	
Mustard, spicy brown	1 tsp.	0	
Mustard, yellow	1 tsp.	0.1	
Parsley, fresh, chopped	1 tbsp.	0.1	

FOOD	PORTION	NET CARBS (G)	COMMENTS
Pesto sauce	1 tbsp.	0.6	
Pickapeppa sauce	1 tsp.	1	
Pickle, dill or Kosher	1 spear	0.5	
Pickle relish	1 tbsp.	3.3	Contains added sugar
Pickle, sweet, midget (2 inches)	1 pickle	1.2	Contains added sugar
Pimento (roasted red pepper)	1 ounce	0.9	
Salsa, green, no added sugar	1 tbsp.	0.5	
Salsa, red, no added sugar	1 tbsp.	0.8	
Sofrito	1 tbsp.	0.5	
Soy sauce	1 tbsp.	1.1	
Soy sauce, tamari	1 tbsp.	0.1	
Spices or spice mixes like curry powder	1 tbsp.	0	Watch for added sugar
Steak sauce	1 tbsp.	2.5	Avoid brands with added sugar
Tabasco or other hot sauce	1 tbsp.	0	
Taco sauce, red	2 tbsp.	1	
Vinegar, balsamic	1 tbsp.	2.7	
Vinegar, cider	1 tbsp.	0.1	
Vinegar, red wine	1 tbsp.	0	
Vinegar, rice (unsweetened)	1 tbsp.	0	
Vinegar, sherry	1 tbsp.	0.9	
Vinegar, white wine	1 tbsp.	1.5	
Wasabi paste	1 tsp.	2	
BEVERAGES (SEE ALSO DAIRY PRODUCTS)			
Broth/bouillon	1 cup	0.7	
Cappuccino, sugar-free mix	3 tbsp.	3	
Cappuccino, instant powder	1 tsp	0.7	
Club soda	8 ounces	0	
Coffee, decaffeinated or decaf, black, no sugar	8 ounces	0.1	
Coconut "dairy" beverage, unsweetened, unflavored	8 ounces	1	

FOOD	PORTION	NET CARBS (G)	COMMENTS
Coconut water, fresh, unsweetened, no added flavors	8 ounces	6.3	
Diet sodas (noncaloric sweeteners)	12 ounces	0	
Seltzer, plain or essence flavored	12 ounces	0	
Sugar-free mixers	12 ounces	0	
Tea, caffeinated or decaf, brewed	8 ounces	0.7	
Tea, herbal (no sugar)	8 ounces	0.5	
Tea, iced, diet, sugar free, with lemon	8 ounces	1	
Tomato juice	4 ounces	4.4	
Vegetable juice "cocktail"	4 ounces	4.3	
Water, tap, spring, filtered, or mineral	8 ounces	0	
ALCOHOLIC BEVERAGES			
Beer, "lite"	12 ounces	5.6	
Beer, low carb	12 ounces	2.5	May vary by brand
Beer, near	12 ounces	13.7	
Bourbon	1 ounce	0	
Champagne	1 ounce	0	
Gin	1 ounce	0	
Rum, dark	1 ounce	0	
Rum, light or white	1 ounce	0	
Scotch and other brown spirits	1 ounce	0	
Sherry, dry	1 ounce	4.7	
Vodka	1 ounce	0	
Wine, red	3.5 ounces	2.6	
Wine, rosé	3.5 ounces	2	
Wine, white, Sauvignon	3.5 ounces	2	
NUTS AND SEEDS			
Almond butter	2 tbsp.	2.7	
Almond paste	1 ounce	12.2	Not recommended; contains added sugar
Almonds, slivered, blanched	2 tbsp.	1.3	
Almonds, whole, raw	24 nuts	2.7	
Brazil nuts, raw	6 nuts	1.4	
Cashew butter	2 tbsp.	8.2	

FOOD	PORTION	NET CARBS (G)	COMMENTS
Cashews, whole, raw or roasted	2 tbsp.	7.6	
Chestnuts, roasted or steamed	6 nuts	24.1	Consume in extreme moderation in later phases
Coconut, fresh or dried, grated, unsweetened	2 tbsp.	0.7	
Hazelnuts (filberts)	2 tbsp.	1.2	
Macadamia nut butter	2 tbsp.	2	
Macadamia nuts, raw or roasted	10 nuts	1.4	
Nutella	2 tbsp.	21	Not recommended; contains added sugar
Peanut butter, crunchy	2 tbsp.	4.3	
Peanut butter, smooth	2 tbsp.	6	
Peanuts, oil roasted	2 tbsp.	1.1	
Peanuts, dry roasted	2 tbsp.	3.8	
Pecans	2 tbsp.	0.6	
Pine nuts (pignoli)	2 tbsp.	1.6	
Pistachios, hulled	2 tbsp.	3	
Pumpkin seeds, hulled	2 tbsp.	1.2	
Sesame seeds	2 tbsp.	0.8	
Soy "nuts" (roasted soy beans)	2 tbsp.	3	
Sunflower seeds, hulled	2 tbsp.	2	
Tahini (sesame paste)	2 tbsp.	5	
Walnuts	12 halves	1.7	
BERRIES AND FRUITS			
Acerola	½ cup	3.2	
Apples, dried	5 rings	18.3	
Apple, fresh	½ medium	10.4	
Applesauce, unsweetened	½ cup	12.4	
Apricots, canned in juice	3 halves	11.6	
Apricots, dried	6 halves	11.6	
Apricots, fresh	3 medium	9.6	
Banana, small	1 fruit	20.4	
Banana chips	1 ounce	14.4	

FOOD	PORTION	NET CARBS (G)	COMMENTS
Banana, freeze dried	1 ounce	23	
Blackberries, fresh	½ cup	3.3	
Blackberries, frozen, unsweetened	½ cup	8.1	
Blueberries, fresh	½ cup	9	
Blueberries, frozen, unsweetened	½ cup	7.3	
Boysenberries, fresh	½ cup	3.1	
Boysenberries, frozen, unsweetened	½ cup	4.6	
Carambola (star fruit), sliced	½ cup	2.1	
Cherimoya	½ cup	11.8	
Cherries, sour, canned in water	½ cup	9.6	
Cherries, sour, fresh	½ cup	8.2	
Cherries, sweet, canned in water	½ cup	12.7	
Cherries, sweet, fresh	½ cup	10.7	
Clementine	1	7.6	
Cranberries, dried	2 tbsp.	5.8	Contains added sugar
Cranberries, raw	½ cup	8	
Cranberry sauce, jellied	2 tbsp.	13.1	Not recommended; contains added sugar
Cranberry sauce, whole berries	2 tbsp.	12.5	Not recommended; contains added sugar
Dates, fresh, Indian	1 whole	5.3	
Figs, dried	1 small	6.5	
Figs, fresh	1 whole	5.3	
Fruit cocktail, in water	½ cup	8.9	
Grapefruit, red or white, fresh	½ medium	8.9	
Grapefruit, canned, sections	½ cup	10.7	
Grapes, green, seedless	½ cup	13	
Grapes, purple Concord	½ cup	7.5	
Grapes, red, seedless	½ cup	13	
Guava, fresh, pieces	½ cup	7.4	
Guava paste	2 tbsp.	12.9	Contains added sugar
Kiwifruit, fresh	1 fruit	8.1	
Kumquat, fresh	4 fruits	7.1	
Lemon juice	2 tbsp.	2	

FOOD	PORTION	NET CARBS (G)	COMMENTS
Lime juice	2 tbsp.	2.4	
Loganberries, frozen	½ cup	5.7	
Loquat, fresh	10 small	16.7	
Lychees, fresh	½ cup	14.5	
Lychees, fresh, whole	10	14.6	
Mango, dried	1 piece	9.5	
Mango, fresh, pieces	½ cup	11.1	
Mango, freeze dried	1 piece	21	
Mango, frozen, unsweetened	½ cup	14	
Melon, cantaloupe, balls	½ cup	6.5	
Melon, cantaloupe, medium (5-inch diameter)	⅛ fruit	5.1	
Melon, Crenshaw, balls	½ cup	4.6	
Melon, honeydew, balls	½ cup	7.3	
Melon, watermelon, balls	½ cup	5.5	
Nectarine, fresh	1 medium	12.6	
Orange, sections	½ cup	8.5	
Orange, navel, whole	1	14.5	
Papaya, dried	1 piece	12.2	
Papaya, fresh	½ small	7.2	
Passion fruit	¼ cup	7.7	
Peaches, dried, halves	2 halves	13.8	
Peach, fresh	1 small	10.5	
Peaches, halves, canned in water	1 half	4.7	
Pears, halves, canned in water	1 half	4.7	
Pear, Bartlett, fresh, medium	1	21.1	
Pear, Bosc, fresh, small	1	18.3	
Persimmon, fresh	½ small	4.1	
Pineapple, chunks, canned in water	½ cup	9.2	
Pineapple, fresh, chunks	½ cup	9.7	
Plantain, fresh, sliced	½ cup	21.9	
Plums, dried (prunes)	3	16.2	
Plums, dried (prunes), canned in heavy syrup	½ cup	28.1	Not recommended; contains added sugar

FOOD	PORTION	NET CARBS (G)	COMMENTS
Plums, fresh	1 small	6.6	
Plums, purple, canned in water	½ cup	12.6	
Pomegranate	¼ fruit	10.4	
Quince	¼ fruit	3.1	
Raisins, golden	1 tbsp.	6.8	
Raisins, seedless	1 tbsp.	6.8	
Raspberries, fresh, whole	½ cup	3.4	
Raspberries, frozen, unsweetened	½ cup	4.4	
Rhubarb, fresh	½ cup	1.7	
Strawberries, fresh, whole	5 large	5.1	
Strawberries, frozen, unsweetened	½ cup	5.2	
Tangerine, fresh	1 small	8.8	
Tangelo, fresh	1 medium	12	
LEGUMES			
Baked beans w/ pork	½ cup	18.3	Not recommended; contains added sugar
Baked beans, vegetarian	½ cup	21.6	Not recommended; contains added sugar
Black bean dip, regular	2 tbsp.	4	
Black bean dip, spicy	2 tbsp.	4	
Beans w/ pork and tomato sauce, canned	½ cup	18.1	Not recommended; contains added sugar
Black/turtle beans, cooked/canned	¼ cup	6.5	
Black-eyed peas, cooked/canned	¼ cup	6.2	
Cannellini beans, cooked/canned	¼ cup	7	
Chickpeas/garbanzos, cooked/canned	¼ cup	10.9	
Cranberry/Roman beans, cooked/canned	¼ cup	5.7	
Falafel	2-ounce patty	18.1	
Fava beans, cooked/canned	¼ cup	5.6	
Great Northern beans, cooked/canned	¼ cup	10.6	
Hummus	2 tbsp.	4.8	
Kidney beans, cooked/canned	¼ cup	5.9	
Lentils, cooked/canned	¼ cup	4	

FOOD	PORTION	NET CARBS (G)	COMMENTS
Lima beans, baby, fresh/frozen, cooked	¼ cup	6.1	
Lima beans, large, cooked/canned	¼ cup	6.1	
Navy beans, cooked/canned	¼ cup	10.1	
Peas, split, cooked/canned	¼ cup	6.3	
Pigeon peas, cooked/canned	¼ cup	5.1	
Pink beans, cooked/canned	¼ cup	9.6	
Pinto beans, cooked/canned	¼ cup	6.4	
Refried beans, canned	¼ cup	6.1	
Soy beans, black, canned	½ cup	0.5	
Soybeans, green (edamame), shelled	¼ cup	1.5	
WHOLE GRAINS			
Barley, hulled, dry	¼ cup	25.8	
Barley, pearl, cooked	½ cup	19.2	
Bulgur, cooked	½ cup	12.8	
Corn meal, dry	2 tbsp.	10.6	
Couscous, cooked	½ cup	17.1	
Couscous, whole wheat, dry	¼ cup	31	
Cracked wheat, dry	¼ cup	24	
Hominy, canned	½ cup	9.7	
Kasha (buckwheat groats), cooked	½ cup	14.5	
Masa (white corn flour)	2 tbsp.	10	
Millet, cooked	½ cup	19.5	
Noodles, egg, cooked	½ cup	19.2	
Noodles, Japanese somen, cooked	½ cup	23.4	
Noodles, rice, dry	1 ounce	24.4	
Noodles, Thai rice, dry	1 ounce	22.3	
Noodles, Udon, dry	1 ounce	18	
Oat bran, raw	2 tbsp.	6	
Oatmeal, rolled, cooked	½ cup	12.1	
Oatmeal, steel cut, raw	¼ cup	11.5	
Pasta, fresh, cooked	3 ounces	20.4	
Pasta, macaroni, protein enriched, cooked	½ cup	20.3	
Pasta, all shapes, cooked	½ cup	16	

FOOD	PORTION	NET CARBS (G)	COMMENTS
Pasta, spinach spaghetti, cooked	½ cup	15.5	
Pasta, whole wheat, cooked	½ cup	15.4	
Pasta, corn, cooked	½ cup	16.2	
Pasta, quinoa, cooked	½ cup	16.3	
Pasta, rice, cooked	½ cup	21	
Pasta, semolina, rigatoni, dry	1 ounce	19.7	
Pasta, sesame rice, cooked	½ cup	16.5	
Pasta, spelt whole grain, elbows, dry	1 ounce	17.4	
Quinoa, cooked	¼ cup	8.6	
Rice, Basmati, dry	¼ cup	35	
Rice, brown, medium grain, cooked	½ cup	21.2	
Rice, short-grain risotto, dry	¼ cup	42.5	
Rice, white, cooked	½ cup	21.9	
Rice, wild, cooked	½ cup	16	
Tabbouleh	¼ cup	20	
Wheat berries, dry	¼ cup	27	
Wheat bran, raw	2 tbsp.	1.6	
Wheat germ, toasted	2 tbsp.	4.9	
BREAD, CRACKERS, TORTILLAS			
Bread, whole wheat pita	1 small	13.3	Check label for white flour and sugar
Bread, pumpernickel	One 1-ounce slice	11.6	Check label for white flour and sugar
Bread, rye	One 1-ounce slice	12.1	Check label for white flour and sugar
Bread, whole grain	One 1-ounce slice	10.2	Check label for white flour and sugar
Bread, whole wheat	One 1-ounce slice	12.6	Check label for white flour and sugar
Crackers, 100% stoned wheat	3 crackers	6.2	
Crackers, brown rice thins	8 crackers	14.1	
Crispbread, Bran-a-Crisp	1 cracker	4	
Crispbread, Finn Crisp	1 cracker	7	
Crisp bread, Kavli Crispy Thin	3 crackers	11	

FOOD	PORTION	NET CARBS (G)	COMMENTS
Crisp bread, Ryvita Flavorful Fiber	2 crackers	11	
Crisp bread, Wasa Hearty Rye	1 cracker	7	
Flatbread, JJ Flats	1 cracker	2.8	
DESSERTS			
Sugar-free gelatin, all flavors	½ cup	0	
Baking chocolate, unsweetened	1 ounce	3.8	
ATKINS NUTRITIONALS			
Atkins Advantage Meal Bars			
Chocolate Chip Cookie Dough	1 bar	3	
Chocolate Chip Granola	1 bar	3	
Chocolate Peanut Butter	1 bar	2	
Cinnamon Bun	1 bar	3	
Cookies n' Crème	1 bar	3	
Mudslide	1 bar	3	
Peanut Butter Granola	1 bar	3	
Peanut Fudge Granola	1 bar	2	
Strawberry Almond	1 bar	3	
Atkins Advantage Snack Bars			
Caramel Chocolate Peanut Nougat	1 bar	3	
Caramel Double Chocolate Crunch	1 bar	4	
Caramel Chocolate Nut Roll	1 bar	3	
Caramel Fudge Brownie	1 bar	3	
Cashew Trail Mix	1 bar	5	
Coconut Almond Delight	1 bar	2	
Dark Chocolate Almond Coconut Crunch	1 bar	3	
Dark Chocolate Decadence	1 bar	4	
Triple Chocolate	1 bar	3	
Atkins Advantage Ready-to-Drink Shakes			
Café Caramel	1 shake	2	
Dark Chocolate Royale	1 shake	2	
French Vanilla	1 shake	1	
Milk Chocolate Delight	1 shake	2	

THE NEW ATKINS FOR A NEW YOU WORKBOOK

FOOD	PORTION	NET CARBS (G)	COMMENTS
Mocha Latte Shake	1 shake	2	
Strawberry	1 shake	1	
Atkins Day Break Bars			
Apple Crisp	1 bar	3	
Cherry Pecan	1 bar	6	
Chocolate Chip Crisp	1 bar	3	
Chocolate Hazelnut	1 bar	3	
Chocolate Oatmeal Fiber	1 bar	7	
Cranberry Almond	1 bar	2	
Peanut Butter Fudge Crisp	1 bar	2	
Vanilla Fruit & Nut	1 bar	5	
Atkins Day Break Ready-to-Drink Shakes			
Creamy Chocolate	1 shake	3	
Strawberry Banana	1 shake	2	
Wild Berry	1 shake	2	
Atkins Endulge Bars			
Caramel Nut Chew	1 bar	2	
Chocolate Caramel Mousse	1 bar	2	
Chocolate Coconut	1 bar	3	
Nutty Fudge Brownie	1 bar	2	
Peanut Butter Cups	1 bar	2	
Peanut Caramel Cluster	1 bar	3	
Atkins Cuisine			
All Purpose Baking Mix	⅓ cup	5	
Penne Pasta	½ cup dry	19	
Atkins Breakast Frozen Meals			
Farmhouse-Style Sausage Scramble	1 tray	5	
Homestyle Waffle Breakfast	1 tray	4	
Tex-Mex Scramble	1 tray	5	
Atkins Entrée Frozen Meals			
Beef Merlot	1 tray	6	
Chicken & Broccoli Alfredo	1 tray	5	
Chile Con Carne	1 tray	4	

FOOD	PORTION	NET CARBS (G)	COMMENTS
Crustless Chicken Pot Pie	1 tray	5	
Italian Sausage Primavera	1 tray	5	
Lemongrass Chicken & Vegetable Hot Pot	1 tray	6	
Meatloaf with Portobello Mushroom Gravy	1 tray	7	
Roasted Turkey with Green Beans	1 tray	6	

THE NEW ATKINS FOR A NEW YOU WORKBOOK